MISSION
IMPROBABLE
How I Healed Bipolar Disorder without Drugs

S. Deborah Fryer

S Deborah Frye

Synergy Books Publishing
U.S.A.

MISSION IMPROBABLE
How I Healed Bipolar Disorder without Drugs

© 2014 S. Deborah Fryer

ISBN: 978-1-936434-59-6

Synergy Books Publishing
www.synergy-books.com

• • •

S. Deborah Fryer

TABLE OF CONTENTS

• • •

MISSION IMPROBABLE

OTHER BOOKS BY THE AUTHOR:

WITH A BRUSH IN MY MOUTH: *The Autobiography of Johannes Michalski*

MISSION IMPROBABLE is available as an e-book on:
Amazon's Kindle & Barnes and Noble's Nook

Additional Copies of Mission Improbable can be ordered at:

missionimpeccablebiographies@gmail.com
Or
Mission Impeccable Books
P.O. Box 112, Basalt ID 83218

S. Deborah Fryer

Praise for
MISSION IMPROBABLE

Deborah Fryer has been a friend of mine for nearly twenty years. She has suffered and triumphed over more hardship than most people I know. Afflicted with bipolar disorder, she has suffered a loveless childhood, a bitter divorce, single parenthood, and almost constant economic struggle. However, even through all that, she has shown an extraordinary ability to heal herself mentally and emotionally without the use of drugs. She has relied instead on nutrition, therapy, prayer forgiveness, loving service to others, a never-say-die attitude, and an unyielding adherence to her faith and moral beliefs. She truly is an amazing woman!

Darrell Smith
Advertising Copywriter
Salt Lake City, Utah

When I first met Deborah Fryer, I left feeling totally inspired. She was one of the most pleasant, confident people I had ever met. Never in a million years would I have guessed

• • •
5

that she came from the devastating depths of depression and mental illness depicted in this book. The process of her healing is truly a miracle considering where she has been, and I can attest that she really has been healed. For anyone who is in the grip of bipolar disorder or depression, this book will give you hope.

Andrew M. Berg
Illustrator

FOREWORD

Happiness can be an elusive thing, even for the best adjusted individuals bustling in the world around us. However, I believe that it is something we all innately aspire to. Certainly, the deck seems stacked against those confronted with the daily obstacles imposed by mental illness.

All too often I see people dealing with mental problems who interpret their personal challenge in finding happiness as a defect in themselves. Their condition turns them into their own worst critics. The trouble with this train of thought is that there is no relief. After all, how can one be happy when he or she is the problem?

Deborah Fryer was one such person. I use the word *was* deliberately and proudly, because I knew her when she was that person. Today, I know a different Deborah-one who no longer believes she is the problem. She has come to see her diagnosis of bipolar disorder for what it is-an obstacle to be overcome, not a life sentence.

Deb has taught me that there is no shortcut to finding happiness. Sometimes we may gather a lot of heartache along the way, but if we have hope and can ask for help, the journey will not be futile. It is a fallacy to think that we need to tackle these challenges alone. I certainly wouldn't trust myself under the hood of my car, so why should I feel the need to trust myself with the burden of all that happens inside my heart and my head? It is never easy to trust, and it is sometimes equally challenging to hope. Still, change or growth cannot happen without these values.

Deborah Fryer has shown me by her actions, and in this beautifully articulated book, how her life is different because she was willing to trust and hope and work. There is no greater tribute I can give her than to say that I know this woman to be one of the most courageous people I have ever met. Her reward is the happiness she lives and breathes.

Kevin Johnson, LCSW
St George, Utah

ACKNOWLEDGEMENTS

My deepest gratitude goes to Anthony Stephan and his family for all they have done, and are doing, on behalf of the mentally ill. I honor them for their loss and sacrifice over the past twenty years.

Great honor goes to David Hardy, a brilliant biologist, for what he has done to contribute to the mental wellness of thousands of people. I look forward to that number becoming millions in the future.

I am indebted to the staff at Truehope Nutritional Support Ltd for their advice and counsel as I came back from the darkest days of my life. Special thanks to Catherine who has been my counselor for the past ten years, and who has given me countless hours of help, advice and comfort.

I would also like to thank the professionals in the field of psychotherapy who gave me the assistance I needed to make lasting changes. Particular and heartfelt thanks to Kevin Johnson, who willingly wrote the foreword despite being supremely busy. He has been my greatest advocate and cheering section, and helped me to see what was really going on in my life. To him I owe a great debt of gratitude.

• • •

Very great thanks to Robert and Rulene Allen for their consistent belief in me, their friendship, love and especially their support and help for this project.

I am grateful to Darrell Smith who has proved a loyal friend and for his great generosity to me and my children.

Many thanks go to Andy and Abbie Berg who gave me a place to write this book, and who reviewed the manuscript.

Thank you also to the Soda Springs library staff, for their encouragement and help during the execution of this project.

Finally, and most importantly, thank you to my children for all they endured at the hands of a very limited, bipolar mother. I know it wasn't easy, but I'm well now, and I continue to love you beyond measure.

S. Deborah Fryer

INTRODUCTION

Two roads converged in a wood and I-
I took the one less traveled by,
And that has made all the difference.

Robert Frost: The Road Not Taken

There is nothing more horrifying than being a prisoner in one's own mind. Today marks eleven years since my prison door began to open.

This is not a medical book. It is a personal history, and an attempt to explain in simple language, what I have suffered, and how I have been healed. I feel a great responsibility to share this information and have endeavored to do so accurately and truthfully.

My own experiences, as well as the experiences of people I've met, have led me to draw certain conclusions, and I take full responsibility for them.

There are no footnotes, no medical terms, and no educated references, despite the fact that I have read many books and articles on the subject. However, I do include a list in the back of a variety of sources of knowledge I have found helpful.

I urge those who may be suffering from any form of mental illness, to be responsible, and to keep taking whatever medications have been prescribed by their physicians. I also urge them to find out for themselves if they are suitable candidates for the approach described herein.

I hope and pray that this little book will help someone, somewhere, to know that there is a way out of that prison, that healing mental illness is not only possible, it is probable.

S. Deborah Fryer
12 February 2014

• • •

CHAPTER ONE

MY SYMPTOMS

Driving down the road from a high school in St George in the fall of 2013, my heart glowed because I knew that I had finally found what I was supposed to be doing in life. I had just spoken to the entire school in the auditorium about never giving up, that you don't have to have any kind of special gift or talent to be successful, and that you just have to work hard and *know* that you can do anything you put your mind to.

I couldn't believe that I had said that. There I was standing on a stage in a spotlight in front of more than a hundred teenagers, who in a former day would have intimidated me, cracking jokes, laughing, positive and cheerful, telling them they could be what they wanted to be.

● ● ●

My journey in life had seemed anything but successful. There were times when I just wanted to kill myself and be done with it. Now here I was, unrecognizable! I prayed all the way home, thanking God for the privilege.

And now, as they say, to the rest of the story..........

I was forty-two in 1996 and had been divorced two years. We had just lost the only home my children had known because of the death of our landlady. I became severely depressed for several weeks and my therapist recommended I see a psychiatrist to be evaluated for some kind of medication. He said he knew I didn't like drugs, but I had to have something to make me better.

My first interview with the psychiatrist ended with him telling me that, had I taken medication at twenty-two-years-old, I wouldn't have suffered all that I had over the past two decades. I had no idea up to that point that I was mentally ill, and that by the time I found a real cure, my illness would span almost a half century.

Shortly after the first drug took effect I remember thinking to myself:

"So this is what it feels like to be happy!"

People don't usually go into a doctor's office to get help for mania. They go when they're depressed; yet they may not know they are suffering from depression. The doctors I saw in my forties could see I was depressed and naturally prescribed anti-depressants. The trouble was, even though I related my life history to them, mania was never discussed or detected. They hadn't seen the bigger picture, and in truth, neither had I. I had no idea what mania was!

From sad experience I now know that an anti-depressant is the wrong prescription for someone who is manic-depressive. It was akin to putting me in an elevator with no ceiling. I just kept going up! I have often wondered whether my recovery would not have been much easier had I never taken anti-depressants.

The doctor told me it would take around six weeks for me to see a lifting of the depression. I actually saw a change in days, and within two weeks I was very happy-too happy. Little did I know at the time that I was manic. I remember dancing around the kitchen with my children, strumming tennis racquets to the sound of "Dizzy Miss Lizzie" by the Beatles. It was so much fun. But the fun didn't last.

Everybody pretty much knows what a depressed person looks like, but mania is harder to discern. When suffering mania I could appear highly entertaining and witty, the life and soul of the party. It could have been mistaken for a personality trait, yet the instability that came with it often went undetected, at least by friends and acquaintances. Family members, however, were a different story. They usually knew there was more going on.

• • •

MISSION IMPROBABLE

Throughout my life I had felt alone in the world, especially in crowds. I was socially awkward and felt isolated. It didn't matter where I was-at school, church, parties, dances or any social gathering-I felt invisible and left out. It was like I was sitting on a fence watching life go by rather than being in it. I was either watching the world or watching myself. I felt disconnected from people. I didn't belong anywhere. I felt unworthy to be around people. I didn't belong to anyone.

I had extreme fear of authority figures. I was very obedient to my parents and teachers because I feared the consequences. Police and government workers scared me as they seemed stern and lacking in humanity. Confident or dominant people and leaders generally, were scary. I compared myself to everyone and always fell short. I was fear based.

When something or someone new came into my life I would become very excited, then after a few weeks, I would lose interest. I would often give up whatever the project or relationship I was in at the time, because I no longer had the reserves of energy for it. I came to the conclusion that nothing lasts, that I would never have any close or long-term friendships, and that ultimately, I could not succeed at anything.

If something bad happened, I would get completely buried in the negative. A simple upset or misunderstanding became a monumental and misery-

• • •

making problem that plunged me into despair. At certain times I thought people liked me, but sometimes I felt I didn't have a friend in the world. I could not control thought processes or impulses. Even though I knew what was right, I couldn't follow through. Impulses overtook me like a rocket going off.

My symptoms varied in intensity and frequency. Either I didn't have them at all, or they were incessant. They were not always noticed or understood by professionals either, so I am going to present a list of symptoms that I recognized over the years that corresponded with my own. I have spoken to many sufferers in the past eleven years and, although there are some variations, a lot of these symptoms are common among people with bipolar disorder.

I'm doing this at the beginning of this book to save people time wondering if this is their problem. I have included every little thing that I experienced, though obviously I cannot rate the degree to which I was affected by each one. I don't intend to discuss them all for fear that this book may never be finished.

I do include them, though, in the hope that they may be helpful. Some groupings are collated under specific headings to make for easier reading. They were compiled at various times, years apart, so there may be some repetition. However, I want to include them all for authenticity.

• • •

SYMPTOMS *(compiled January 2001, two years before I suspected bipolar disorder. Therefore the heading MANIC has been added.)*

DEPRESSIVE

- Very lethargic; don't want to do anything
- Don't want to think about anything
- No interest in anything; could care less
- Feel that I have nothing
- Leave me alone signals sent out to other people
- Uninterested in others
- Can't focus mentally
- Can't follow through with goals and plans
- Terrified to act
- Can't finish projects
- Can't act on plans made
- Reclusive and don't want to leave the house
- Very overwhelmed
- Exhausted
- Don't want to talk
- Very pessimistic
- Unfeeling

- Hopeless and overwhelmed about the future
- Needy and dependent
- All or nothing thinking

MANIC *(To those who have not experienced mania, this list may not seem unusual, and may not be seen as being a problem. It must be emphasized that many of these symptoms should probably be prefaced with the word "excessive.")*

- Outgoing, friendly, sociable and loud
- Dominate conversations; talk over other people
- High functioning and achieve a lot in a day
- Inspired with lots of ideas
- Makes goals; planning and dreams constantly
- Elated and excitable
- Strong feelings and passionate about things
- Altruistic and giving
- Creative thinker and educator
- Detailed list making
- Adventurous and courageous; risk taker
- Start many projects, but can't finish
- Create charts and plans
- Very productive
- Very busy and active
- Excessively talkative
- Critical, fault-finding and judgmental

● ● ●

- Demanding and controlling
- Raging bull
- Risqué humor
- Arrogant and disrespectful
- Super optimistic
- Very encouraging and helpful
- Warm and softhearted
- Service oriented
- Can become suddenly mean and hateful
- Overly detail oriented
- Can achieve just about anything
- Don't need anything or anyone
- Workaholic
- Excessively long, deliberate focus which can last hours
- Euphoria
- Excessive emotion; drama queen

SYMPTOMS *(Compiled from various sources as well as noticed in self-January 2003)*

DEPRESSION

- Sad, anxious, empty mood lasting weeks
- Loss of interest in all activities

- Feelings of hopelessness and guilt
- Feel everything I do is pointless and worthless
- Uninterested in food or cooking
- Feel exhausted and slowed-down
- Frequent, daily thoughts of suicide, death and dying
- Feel alone in crowds and groups
- Don't want to be seen in daylight
- Don't want to meet people in passing or unexpectedly
- Avoiding people
- Repeated doubts
- Don't want to answer phone or make phone calls
- Don't like people coming to house unannounced

MANIA
- Very talkative and feel like I am vomiting words
- Excessive talking on the phone
- Joke and story telling
- Center of a crowd entertaining them
- Pressure to write and make lists

• • •

- Starting multiple projects and not able to finish them
- A multitude of ideas streaming through my mind
- Excessively interested and opinionated in a lot of subjects
- Out of control thinking and intrusive thoughts
- Extremely irritated and agitated

PANIC

- Racing heartbeat
- Have to get out of a place or go somewhere immediately!
- Dizziness and lightheadedness
- Flushes and chills
- Feelings of unreality
- Feel out of control and crazy
- Fear of dying of various illnesses
- Fear crowds, machines, driving a car, loud noises, speed and fast-paced activities
- Afraid to leave the house
- Fear of the unknown
- Feel like about to have a heart attack

• • •

OBSESSIVE/COMPULSIVE
- Constant house cleaning and organizing
- Fixated on certain thoughts and ideas
- Need for symmetry and order
- Aggressive impulses
- Constant need for change, variety and stimulation
- Requesting and demanding assurances
- Arranging and rearranging furniture, papers etc.

SOCIAL ANXIETY
- Excessive persistent fear of my performance being judged
- Afraid of meeting new people as well as people I already know
- Not comfortable eating in front of people
- Afraid to speak in social situations
- Sick with fear of tests and filling in forms
- Afraid of being questioned or any kind of scrutiny
- Sweating and muscle tension in company

• • •

- Not interested in a social life
- Feeling very awkward in social situations
- Terrified of authority figures
- Feeling unattractive to the opposite sex

MY SYMPTOMS *(Catalogued and sent in a letter to my sister so my siblings could see if they could relate - October 2004)*

- General depression from early childhood throughout adulthood
- Suicidal thoughts from puberty throughout adulthood
- Extreme loneliness and inability to socialize
- Feeling alone in crowds
- Unrealistic thinking and delusions of grandeur
- Extremely low self-image
- Self-hate
- No self-confidence
- Feeling alone and disconnected from everyone, including family members
- Feeling like I had no power or control over my life
- Feeling that nothing would ever change or be better

• • •

- Feeling destined to have a hard and terrible life, that nothing would improve
- Feeling hopeless and helpless about personal problems
- Feeling unloved and unlovable
- Unable to make or keep friends or any kind of close relationships
- Excessive cleaning and ordering of possessions
- Scared to use machines e.g. car, computer, typewriter, sewing machine
- Excessive spending; adrenaline rush from shopping
- Re-organizing furniture and moving rooms around in house
- Excessive talking and phoning people
- Excessive writing and pressure to read and write
- Extreme irritability, anger and rage as years passed
- Inability to work outside the home or in stressful jobs
- As I got older, became less able to function even at home
- Seeking constant change by moving from place to place
- Constant need to keep busy; unable to sit still; driven

• • •

- Sleep problems; unable to fall asleep, stay asleep and waking early
- Brilliant thoughts and insights
- Very quick and incisive mind
- Too much thinking
- Hard time focusing
- Excessive planning and goal setting but things never came to fruition
- Starting tasks and projects with great enthusiasm, but never finishing any
- Bored easily and very impatient
- Hard to feel empathy
- Always felt very immature; not really grown up; related better with younger people, but not peer group
- Dependent personality; wanted to be rescued from my hard life
- Inability to follow recipes, plans, maps and other written instructions; written details made me anxious
- Fear of learning new things, especially subjects in school; overwhelmed mentally and had a hard time making the shift to learning new information
- Fearful and overwhelmed by the Internet because of massive amount of information

• • •

- Extreme need to share learned information and ideas
- Problems with food e.g. tastes and textures
- Eating seemed like a waste of time, a chore which got in the way of me doing things
- Constant health problems; stomach aches, headaches, earaches, migraines, backaches, leg aches and complaining about body problems
- Trouble understanding consequences of words or actions
- Out of touch with reality; creating a big dream; thinking I'm invisible
- Feeling invincible, like nothing can touch or harm me
- Superior attitude; thinking nobody understands the things I understand
- Panic attack
- Severe anxiety
- Obsessed with details on the one hand, but overwhelmed by them on the other
- Hard to make even small decisions
- Going from elation to despair in the same day
- Extreme tiredness
- Afraid to be away from home for very long periods of time

• • •

SYMPTOMS COMPILED AFTER 10 YEARS ON TRUEHOPE PROGRAM *(I include these symptoms which I wrote as a well person.)*

- Anxiety in almost every situation, even doing simple tasks at home, when nobody was watching
- Obsessive thoughts and behavior
- Excessive worrying
- Feeling spaced out
- Massive insecurity
- Feeling empty and alone, like in a bubble all by myself
- Difficulty making friends because it was too much work; felt I didn't have the emotional reserves to start relationships or invest the time and energy in them to keep them going
- Tendency to isolate
- Difficulty joining in group activities
- Negative self-talk
- Negative self-view
- Brooding
- Resentful
- Angry

• • •

- Loss of authentic feelings, especially with the use of psychotropic medications
- Going from hating spending money to excessive shopping
- Credit card debt; hard to curb spending or anticipate the consequences of debt
- Hated my own reflection in mirrors
- Disliked my photo being taken
- Wanted change, but didn't cope well with it
- Wanting to be on the move traveling by bus, train, plane etc.
- Risk taking to the extreme
- Daily suicidal thoughts
- Overeating and starvation depending on mood
- Constantly worried about others watching and judging me
- Perfectionism
- Excessive judging of others
- Fearful of every situation no matter how benign
- Feelings of being unloved
- Possessive; wanting a person to be my close friend and wanting them to have me as their only friend

- Catastrophizing
- Giving power to dangerous people
- Remaining in bad situations for years
- No trust of others
- Had to be independent; scared to ask for help
- Nightmares
- Nervous and easily frightened
- Constantly upset by what was going on around me
- Sad and unhappy
- Pressure to write, to make lists, journal entries and write letters
- Excessive reading; feeling so involved in a book, such as a novel, that I felt bereft when it ended and I had to come back to reality
- While watching a movie I felt like I was the main character and that I wanted to be him or her
- Very weak boundaries with people who could do me serious harm
- Feeling desperate after certain periods spent alone
- Dark feelings of hopelessness

• • •

CHAPTER TWO

MY ANCESTORS

All I know about my family history came from my mother's lips, and I have no idea whether any of it is true. I am assuming that it is, and am only including it to show the kind of chaos I was born into.

My mother hated her father, and my dad hated his mother. Therefore, I was raised without extended family, even though they lived within five miles of our house.

My mother told me that her father was a drinking man. That was the terminology in those days for an alcoholic. In 1959, eight years after she had severed her relationship with him, he won the football pools. His total

• • •

winnings were the equivalent of a million dollars in today's money. At the same time his doctor warned him that he had a blood clot near his heart and that if he continued drinking, it would kill him. This confirms to me that his drinking was not merely social, if his doctor was aware of it. He actually lived till he was eighty-one, and didn't stop drinking.

My mother described him as a womanizer, unfaithful to my sick grandmother who had epilepsy. She told me he had been having an affair with another woman since she, my mother, was twelve-years-old. When her mother died at age fifty, after falling into the fire during a seizure, he moved his mistress in with him. My mother was nineteen. (I recently discovered from one of my mother's cousins who found me on the internet, that my grandparents were actually separated when my mother was twelve.)

One day my mother went to school without her pencil box. She went home at lunchtime to get it, and as she turned the corner of the street, she was met with a sickening sight. The dustbin men were throwing her Old English sheepdog Sadie, whom she adored, onto the dust cart, dead. She said that she knew her father had killed it. I have often wondered if he was jealous of her relationship with the dog, and if Sadie was her protector against him.

I once asked my mother about my grandfather's behavior towards her, and she angrily retorted that he had never laid a hand on her! She was very emphatic about it

● ● ●

and it took me by surprise. I question this statement because her father was apparently a violent man.

When I was twenty my mother told me that she gave birth to a child out of wedlock when she was my age. She said her father told her that she either give the baby up for adoption, or she would be put out on the street. Interestingly enough, he apparently got a girl pregnant in his youth, but escaped his responsibilities by joining the army, going off to India and leaving the young woman to deal with the consequences.

My mother told me the circumstances surrounding her pregnancy, the name of the father, and how he had abandoned her while the wedding was being planned. In those days, even my mother's friends crossed the street when they saw her pregnant and unmarried. I don't know what her relationship with her mother was like, but it must have been a shock when she died before the baby was born. The child was adopted by a family living not far away, so my mother was allowed to continue living at home. She told me she was treated like Cinderella by the woman who had taken her mother's place.

While doing some family history research a few years ago I decided to find my uncle, my mother's brother, who was four years her junior. My uncle wrote to me and I also spoke to him on the phone. He told me that my mother was very angry and mean as a child and teenager, and that he didn't like her. He said that she left home when she was about fourteen to live with a friend and her family, and that he was glad to see the back of her. I had assumed my mother lived at home during her entire teenage years. Now that I know my grandparents were separated, I wonder which of her parents she lived with. Maybe she returned to her father's house when she found out she was pregnant, because she had nowhere else to go.

A few months after the baby was adopted she met my dad and was soon pregnant again. They had to marry quickly, and twelve children were born to them in eighteen years. I was the second of that twelve. We were all premature, two were stillborn, and one, twin to a stillborn brother, lived only a few hours.

Just after her father won the football pools my mother was at the funeral of one of her relatives. Her father was there with his mistress on his arm. Someone came up to her and asked if she was going to talk to him because, after all, he was a wealthy man now. My mother said she didn't care how much money he had, she wanted nothing to do with him. She would not see him again until he was on his deathbed, and when she arrived with most of her children, he thought she was from the Catholic Church, which he had joined later in life. He did not even know he was grandfather to her nine children. Apparently he had given most of his money to the church.

I don't know too much about my mother's older brother. She told me he was a glass blower and also a heavy drinker. She had no relationship with him as an adult either. I never met any of my cousins, although everyone lived within a few miles of our house. I could have run into them in town and never have known them.

My mother also told me that she had an uncle who had hung himself after his daughter accused him of molesting her. The family my mother married into had the same kinds of problems-infidelity, alcoholism and promiscuity.

I know very little about my mother's mother and her family. Many years ago I received a letter from someone who knew her personally, who told me my grandmother had been a very depressed woman, a sad and lonely figure.

I have studied bipolar disorder thoroughly over the past decade, and it is obvious to me that my mother's family was beset by the illness. From what my mother described, I believe her father, at the very least, was also afflicted with it. I can only guess at the rest.

● ● ●

MISSION IMPROBABLE

CHAPTER THREE

THIS CAN'T BE MY LIFE!

Some of my earliest childhood memories are from my pre-school years. I remember as a toddler feeling anxious and lonely. I was extremely fearful, especially of loud noises, crowds, getting hurt physically and authority figures.

I spent hours sitting at the hearth in front of a roaring fire, watching the flames flickering in the grate. I didn't always like going out to play because when I was outdoors, I often felt disoriented. The warm fire helped me to feel better. So did being in water, which I found soothing and calming. I developed a love of swimming, having warm baths, walking near lakes, ponds and fountains, and being out in the rain, splashing in puddles.

• • •

It was hard for me to think of my mother's house as a home, as there was no safety there; no soft place to fall. I craved a cozy, comforting place, but my mother's house was anything but that.

I had no idea when I was a child that my mother was mentally ill. I didn't understand why she was constantly upset, shouting, screaming and punishing us. She raged over little things of no consequence. We were slapped, punched, kicked, beaten with belts and canes, shoes and hairbrushes. She pulled hair, smacked faces, used a belt on bare legs and bottoms, and banged heads on walls.

As a child I never acted like a girly girl, and didn't feel particularly feminine. As I entered puberty, I used to think I ought to have been a boy. I have never had a desire to do really masculine activities, but I liked being around boys more than girls. I found boys easier to talk to and to understand. I thought girls were mean and petty, but I was still interested in girls' activities. I liked dressing up in high heels and playing with dolls. I did have an unusually deep voice, though, even as a two-year-old and neighbors even remarked on it.

Following is a sample of incidents that colored my childhood. There were many more, often involving my other siblings. Some of these punishments were carried out in front of neighbors and friends. I include them merely to show the kinds of things my mother did on a daily basis. These things have been forgiven and forgotten by me now,

• • •

but they were a source of great pain and suffering for many years.

One example of her mistreatment was when I was at home one day feeling unwell. I was about nine or ten, and not sick enough to be in bed. My mother had a predictable routine when she was not working outside the home. She would do her housework and food preparation in the morning, and then socialize in the afternoons. This usually involved going over to a neighbor's house and chatting over tea, cigarettes and knitting.

On this particular day, she asked me if I would like to earn sixpence by polishing the dining table and chairs while she was out. This involved using liquid furniture polish that had to be applied with one cloth and buffed with another. It was a big table with bulbous legs, and the chairs had solid wooden backs. It was a big job for a child and took me almost the whole afternoon.

When she came back, she saw that I had used over half the bottle of polish, and she immediately went into a rage. She knocked me to the cold, linoleum-covered floor and began kicking me in the stomach with her shoes on. She shouted and swore at me, telling me that if I cried or made a sound, she would do worse.

I don't know how long I lay alone on the floor after she left the room, but I remember going into a state of shock and unreality. All I wanted to do was to disappear,

● ● ●

die, or run away-but there was nowhere to go. I never did get my sixpence.

Another incident happened when I was even younger, about five or six. On many occasions I was sent to the corner shop to get a loaf of bread or something. Mr. Chadwick's was a general grocer shop with a high counter that dwarfed most adults. As a little child I would get lost in the queue, waiting for what seemed like an eternity to be served. I'd get bored, and was usually hungry, so I started helping myself from the tins of biscuits that lined the front of the counter. They had glass lids and you could see the contents clearly. My weakness was for chocolate biscuits. Of course I was a child and didn't even think to hide the chocolate smears on my little hands and face.

The next time I went to the shop was with my older sister. Mr. Chadwick told her to inform my mother what I had been doing. I was so afraid to go home. When she heard what I had done, my mother grabbed a leather belt from its nail on the wall, dragged me into the street, and proceeded to thrash me all the way to the shop and back. Chadwick's shop was a good block and a half away. I could see that the shop owner was sorry he had said anything, and was disturbed at the way my mother was treating me. When I went to school on Monday, one of my teachers pulled me aside and asked how I got the bruises on my legs. I said nothing even when she showed them to another teacher. Nothing was ever done about it.

• • •

I had no idea that I was depressed as a child, but I was constantly being told to cheer up, that it might never happen. I was upset every time someone said that to me. I had no idea that I was so morose. My mother told me it was because I was born old that I was so serious. On the other hand, I remember as a teenager having bouts of silliness. I would become the life of the party, cracking jokes and laughing till I cried. I also had an acerbic wit, and my tongue was like a sharp sword if I was crossed.

I was a latch-key kid from the age of nine, and required to do chores and childcare that were similar both in number and detail to what an adult would do. I was also expected to perform well in school. I was at the top of my class in the elementary years and found the work easy. Grammar school, which I entered at eleven-years-old, was a different story. I started having serious difficulty. I now believe this was because I had entered puberty, and my brain was struggling, along with my hormones.

At twelve, I started to dream of my escape from my mother. Throughout my teens I felt increasingly unhappy and unable to cope. I was anxiety-ridden as I tried to meet her exacting standards. I felt overwhelmed by my responsibilities, and the chaos in the family, and became increasingly withdrawn.

As a teenager I had a hard time getting boys to notice me. They just didn't seem interested in me. The few relationships I had with boys didn't last and I always ended

• • •

up heartbroken. Conversely, some boys, even the very good-looking ones, didn't interest me. I wanted to date boys I could talk to. I needed to have deep and interesting conversations with them, to feel connected.

I spent a lot of time alone in my room and became a reading machine with a voracious appetite for knowledge. I always had a book in my hand, which angered my mother more. Reading was a means of escape for me. In high school I read English authors like Jane Austen and Thomas Hardy, as well the works of Russian authors Solzhenitsyn, Turgenev, Dostoevsky and Tolstoy, and French writers like Flaubert, Zola and Balzac. I was very smart and soaked up knowledge like a sponge. After school I excitedly shared what I learned each day with my parents. That was the only way I felt accepted by my mother. She wanted me to do well because she was allowed to stay in school.

While researching bipolar disorder, I discovered that people suffering from this illness tend to be above average intelligence. Apparently, the great appetite for knowledge in those who are bipolar is due to the excess of electrical impulses flowing through the brain, causing pressure to learn, to read, to write and to talk. I was constantly looking for meaningful, mental stimulation. At the same time I was trying to figure out what was real and true in the world.

Although I loved learning I didn't like school much, at least not high school. I was stressed by all the rules, and

• • •

intimidated by the archaic, cold and impersonal atmosphere of the grand old English buildings. I didn't fit in with any particular crowd. I knew everybody and everybody knew me, but I never felt like I really belonged.

By eighteen I had become pretty hopeless, and although I had no desire whatsoever to become a career woman, I settled on becoming a teacher. I moved three hundred miles away from my family to a teacher training college, where I majored in fine arts.

My parents didn't want me to go so far away to college and my relationship with them really deteriorated even further after I left. I felt somehow that leaving was a betrayal of the family, and I was never really accepted back in. I was a big disappointment to them. No matter what I did, I couldn't seem make them happy, or to keep the relationship going. I felt unwanted, and every time I returned for a visit, it ended badly. I was rarely invited for the holidays, and my visits to my family became fewer and fewer.

At college, I found life increasingly austere, although I attended a college in a beautiful country setting. I was by then only an average student, and I struggled to keep up. I now know this was due to depression. I had been drawing seriously since I was ten-years-old and I see now that I used this talent as a sort of occupational therapy, much as my mother used knitting.

● ● ●

MISSION IMPROBABLE

I loved painting and my professors thought I was a good candidate to stay on after graduation to do a bachelors' degree, but I didn't want to stay in school any longer. I was too overwhelmed mentally and emotionally by then and didn't think I was good enough to make a career out of art. I stopped painting and drawing altogether at the age of twenty-six.

The austerity and loneliness I felt at college led me into an early marriage which didn't last. I gave birth to a stillborn child at eight months pregnant, and it was at this juncture that I knew my life was in serious trouble. I had a nervous breakdown and plunged into a year-long depression. I couldn't work, and became isolated from all the people who had been my friends before the baby died.

I became increasingly lonely and though I craved the company of people on the one hand, I was too unhappy and anxious to be around anyone on the other. I had no help or therapy at that point, and doubted that I would ever be able to cope with life again.

I didn't become a school teacher when I left college. I couldn't handle the job interview process. I decided instead to do elderly care and housecleaning, because it was less demanding and stressful. I moved house regularly in order to get away from strained relationships, and to start over when things got too difficult. I was always hoping that the next house, or the next friend,

• • •

S. Deborah Fryer

or the next job, would make a difference to how I felt; but that never happened.

I hitchhiked a lot in my twenties. I was poor and couldn't afford the train or bus fare when I did visit my family. I mostly hitchhiked alone; unaware of the serious risk I was taking. It's a wonder I'm still alive to tell about it. I was oblivious to the dangers in the world.

A year after the stillbirth of my daughter, I decided to move to London, and was soon working seven days a week, sometimes twelve hours a day. I became a workaholic. I had no satisfaction in my life other than work. Work became my new escape. The more I worked, the less time I had to spend alone.

No matter what I did in my twenties, I never felt better. I couldn't reach out to anyone, and nobody reached out to me. I now know I was in a terrible brain fog which was isolating me more and more. During that decade I did a lot of interesting work and met a lot of people, but I never really felt like part of anything. I always felt alone, no matter how many people were around me.

I craved the security of a home and a family. All I wanted was to create an environment of peace and security, filled with love, light and warmth, but that never happened either. I had no security or safety, no roots and no anchor. I was a very needy adult because of the treatment I suffered as a child. Every time a friendship or

● ● ●

relationship went bad, I was distraught and depressed. I just wanted to belong to someone.

I have come to understand through the process of healing, that healthy people are more likely to attract healthy people, and that unhealthy people are more likely to form relationships with unhealthy people. I was not aware when I was in relationships with men that this was the case, and always believed that I was the problem. Now that I am recovered from mental illness, I see that they were all having similar problems to my own.

Now that I know my mother was bipolar, I understand her thinking, feelings and behavior. As I came to know the extent of my mother's suffering through my own, forgiveness was easy. My mother went through it all with only tranquilizers to calm her, and they obviously didn't work. She had no therapy or any other kind of psychiatric help. I could tell she preferred working outside the home, which she did for most of her life. I think family relationships were too hard and demanding emotionally.

In the eighteen years I spent living under my parents' roof I was led to believe that I was the problem. My mother never showed me any love, kindness, warmth or affection. I had no concept of feeling accepted or wanted in my family. I felt basically good for nothing, except for the service I performed cooking and cleaning, washing and ironing, errand running and child care.

• • •

On my thirty-first birthday my mother finally put into words what I had always suspected she felt about me. She flew into a rage and put her hands around my throat. I looked deep into her eyes and told her to go ahead. She pushed me away and slammed off into the living room. I followed her and in tears said:

"You've never loved me have you?" to which she replied:

"You? Who could love you?"

I walked out into the snow that day and never went back. I didn't see her until thirteen years later. This time, she was in her casket.

MISSION IMPROBABLE

CHAPTER FOUR

IT'S IN HER GUT!

I was sick regularly as a child. There always seemed to be something wrong with me. My mother called me a "creaking gate" because I suffered headaches, leg aches, ear aches and general malaise. I just never really felt that well.

Our old family doctor once told her:

"I think it's in her gut!" His words turned out to be prophetic.

• • •

MISSION IMPROBABLE

I had a healthy appetite and ate pretty much anything that was put in front of me, but was always small and thin. I weighed 105lbs my entire teenage and adult life, and for my 5'2" frame, that is considered perfect on English weight charts. I attributed my remaining the same weight for years to having a fast metabolism, and my body utilizing everything I put in my mouth. Little did I know that I was having chronic digestive problems.

I had to write an essay in elementary school about what we ate in our family. I remember the look of chagrin on my parents' faces when I told them I thought our diet was unhealthy, and that we shouldn't be eating white bread. By the time I was twenty and had full control of the food going into my mouth, my eating habits bore little resemblance to those with which I was raised. I became a vegetarian, and drank a lot of milk and orange juice, but still didn't feel any better.

When I gave birth to my stillborn daughter, I felt strongly that her death was in some way related to my eating habits, though the attending physician at the birth contradicted this. This great loss had a shocking impact on me, and I had a nervous breakdown. I returned to my parents' house in Yorkshire to recover, and was prescribed an anti-depressant by our family doctor. When I told him I didn't believe in drugs, he said if I didn't take it, he would put me in a psych unit.

• • •

The drug had a terrible effect on me. I felt like a dead person walking. I had absolutely no feelings, good or bad. I knew I could not continue to take it, and after ten days, I threw the pills away. My mother was furious. One day she found me in tears in the bathtub only days after my loss, and told me coldly to "get over it." I knew that if I was going to get well, I would have to do it on my own. I returned to my flat in Bath three hundred miles away, and started to rebuild my life.

Within a few weeks I adopted the macrobiotic diet, a regimen based on whole grains. My family thought I was crazy, but I stuck with it for eleven years. When I began eating natural foods I gained physical strength like I had not known before. At the age of twenty-five, the year after I lost my daughter, I was swimming twenty-five laps of an Olympic-sized swimming pool every morning. I began doing yoga and other exercises, and I walked everywhere. I learned shiatsu therapy and reflexology and did everything I could to educate myself in eastern medicine. I even got involved in teaching natural foods cooking classes, and eventually started my own natural foods catering and fermented pickle business.

At age twenty-six I moved to London so I could have a fresh start. Although I loved Bath, it was a tourist city and there wasn't much steady work. I knew London would have more opportunities. Though I was daunted at the prospect of big city life, I rose to the challenge, and soon found my way around on my bicycle.

Within a short time I was working seven days a week. I didn't understand about stress in those days, and in time I became exhausted. My depression, anxiety and obsessive tendencies, increased, and I felt more alone than ever. I was okay around people at work for the most part, but I resisted a social life because I felt so awkward. I didn't know what to say, how to do small talk. I still didn't understand that I was having serious mental and emotional problems. It just seemed normal to me to be unhappy and to have to struggle through life.

Finally at the age of twenty-seven I'd had enough of my life the way it was. I sold everything and told my friends I was going to change my life if it was the last thing I did. I bought a one-way ticket to Boston, Massachusetts and traveled across the entire American continent for a year. My life did change during that trip, in a way I had never envisioned. It changed spiritually.

I returned to London, and worked for another four years in my own cleaning business, and worked part-time in an office for a year. Out of the blue I got the opportunity to do some elementary school teaching, which I did for two years.

In 1987 I spent the summer in Provo, Utah, with a view to studying there. The July heat hit me like a ton of bricks. I had never experienced weather over a hundred

• • •

degrees before. My appetite was poor the entire two months of my stay and I drank a lot of water, but when I returned to England my weight had dropped to 98lbs. I was a little concerned, but thought I'd probably put it right back on. I didn't.

I returned to Provo to go to school in 1988 and was married within the year. I immediately became pregnant, and my daughter was born a month prematurely in 1989. I weighed only 125lbs at eight months' gestation, and after her birth it didn't take long for my body to shed the excess weight. I hoped I would bottom out at 105lbs, but I soon returned to 98lbs.

Another two children came in rapid succession. My husband wanted nothing to do with a healthy lifestyle, and I had no choice but to revert to a meat and potatoes diet. I slept only four hours a night, and after four years of abuse, and a two year separation, my marriage ended in divorce.

People would comment regularly on how thin I was. It was hurtful to me-just like being called fat. Some people asked me why I didn't put weight on. I felt like a criminal, as if I was starving myself on purpose. I had a good appetite so I didn't understand why I was so thin.

All this was upsetting for another reason; my mother, who was 5'4" tall weighed 90lbs her entire life. She had twelve pregnancies, but never retained an ounce of weight after the deliveries. She looked like a bird, and on

● ● ●

the one or two occasions I was allowed to hug her, she felt like a skeleton. I was so afraid I was becoming like her.

At thirty-eight years old while nursing my seven-month-old son, I started having hot flashes. My doctor told me I was in early menopause. He thought that the shock of my marriage breaking down was the cause, but I remembered my mother had entered menopause around forty. It lasted until the summer of 2000.

I had moved that year with my children to Medford, Oregon, in a bid to put distance between me and my ex-husband. As the years went by, his behavior towards me escalated, and I had no choice but to move away.

One hot night in our new house, I went to bed with a flat stomach, and in the morning awoke with a belly that resembled a large bowl of Jell-O. I went straight to the doctor who said he had seen the same condition in many middle-aged women. He had no further explanation for it.

I thought it had something to do with my reproductive system because of the menopause coming to an end. I now believe that this condition was related to my gut. I had been under severe stress for twelve years, one of the causes of leaky gut syndrome, which I was eventually to discover I was suffering from.

I was not successful in returning completely to macrobiotics after the divorce. I was too poor to afford to eat many of the foods I needed. Back in the 1970s it had been cheaper to eat natural foods than processed, and

• • •

although I had been able to buy grains and beans in bulk in a Provo food co-op, there were many other products that I just could not obtain.

I struggled on, trying to feel better through diet, but never succeeded. As my children became teenagers, I pretty much gave up. They wanted what their friends ate anyway, so I ended up eating pizza, meat and spaghetti, and fewer and fewer vegetables.

At fifty-years-old I had a gall bladder attack out of nowhere, and had to have it removed. It was a big shock to me. I'd had my tonsils and wisdom teeth removed when I was young, but I never dreamed I would ever have a major surgical procedure. The doctor showed me an x-ray of my gall bladder. There were only a few small stones in the bottom of it. I was surprised, because in photos I had seen of diseased gall bladders, they were completely stuffed with stones. I asked him if I had done the right thing having mine removed, and he told me yes, that he had found it completely lacerated.

Doctors may label surgeries routine procedures, but they are not routine for the patient. My studies in eastern medicine taught me that each organ is inter-dependent, and that there were consequences for removing any of them. The loss of my gall bladder added to the serious downturn in my digestive health.

After the surgery I had to take digestive enzymes and a homeopathic remedy to settle my stomach. I couldn't even put food in my mouth without pain. I stayed away from fats for a long time, knowing that my liver would have to work overtime to digest them properly. It took a long time for my digestive system to seem normal again, and there were many foods I just could not eat any more.

In my mid-fifties I started having a dull pain on the left side of my abdomen which was always there. It wasn't too bad, so I ignored it for a year. Eventually I became really exhausted. It took all the energy I had to go to work. I would come home and lie down on the couch because my legs hurt so much. My ankles became very swollen, even in the morning when I woke up, which was unusual. I discovered I had diverticulosis.

Raising teenage boys meant I had to buy more meat for them. They were developing muscles and craving animal food. I didn't have the energy to make two different meals, and couldn't afford it either, so I would generally eat what they did. Although I knew that a woman in her fifties doesn't need the same kind of nutrition as a teenage boy, I still kept eating the food I prepared for them.

As my health became critical, I knew I would need to make radical changes if things were going to improve. I began practicing something called food combining. This meant I had to separate protein from carbohydrates in the same meal. At first I had no idea what I was doing.

I began by eating a large serving bowl of green salad every lunch time, cutting out all animal food at first.

• • •

Eventually, I would add a couple of ounces of chicken or tuna or steak. I stopped all canned fruit and ate only fresh fruit, by itself, and never with a meal. I ate meat with salad or non-starchy vegetables, not with potatoes or pastry crust. If I had pizza it was vegetarian style. If I wanted mashed potatoes and gravy, I ate them with just vegetables. Beans, which are classified as a carbohydrate, were eaten only with vegetables, never with meat.

Within a week I was feeling better; the pain in the left side of my abdomen diminished and the swelling in my legs went away. In a month my energy was back to normal. Actually, it was better than normal, so I continued to eat this way to try to maintain my intestinal health. An added bonus of food combining was that, over a two-year period, I lost all the excess weight which I had gained from psychotropic medications.

The last anti-depressant I was prescribed drastically altered my metabolism. During the first eight months I was taking it, I put on forty pounds. When I questioned my doctor he said it was no problem and that I looked fine. My weight had increased on other medications so that by the time I was forty-seven I was 117lbs. In eight months on the new drug my weight shot up to 162.5lbs! I looked and felt horrible, but my doctor said I was fine. I didn't feel fine, especially as I didn't have the energy to carry around an extra fifty extra pounds.

● ● ●

MISSION IMPROBABLE

By October 2011, using this method, I returned to my original weight of 105lbs. This was done with zero exercise and not on purpose. I felt better than I had done in years, and even bought a swimsuit! I have heard many middle-aged people say that they cannot lose weight. I've known seniors who are walking, running, cycling and swimming and cannot lose a pound. I really believe that the most important factor is what we put in our mouths. I didn't set out to lose weight, just to heal from diverticulosis. The weight loss was literally a by-product of the food combining.

My joy at being slim again didn't last when my weight kept decreasing. Then I developed pain in my upper abdomen after eating. By Christmas I didn't want to eat at all, but I had planned an English-style Christmas, and baked dozens of mince pies and jam tarts. I noticed that every time I ate pastry, or any carbohydrates, I felt awful. Pastry had always been one of my favorite foods as a child. It was comfort food to me. Not anymore.

In January 2012, I visited an old friend for a few days. She had cured herself of Hodgkin's Lymphoma by eating a raw food diet. I took my own food with me because I knew there was no way I could eat raw food in the winter. At lunchtime she offered me a big green salad full of sprouts and raw chips. I found it surprisingly delicious and very satisfying. While I was eating it, I looked over at my bowls of brown rice and miso soup and told her I didn't

• • •

want to eat that food any more. I ate raw food the entire time I stayed with her and felt somewhat better when I left.

Reluctantly, in late January, as my weight continued to decline and the pain in my abdomen persisted, I went to the doctor. She sent me to the hospital for a whole panel of blood tests and a CT scan. The hospital found nothing wrong. When I went back to the doctor for the results, I commented to her that my symptoms and weight loss reminded me of my mother's lifelong battle. She quipped:

"Well, you can thank your lucky stars that you're only getting it now!" and sent me home to "keep doing what you're doing". At that point I was living on salads because raw food was all I could digest. I weighed 100lbs.

Winter turned to spring and I felt like I was starving. People looking at me must have thought I was anorexic. One day I was talking to someone who had seen my symptoms in other people. He told me I was allergic to gluten! I was shocked. I'd met other people who said they were gluten intolerant, and I thought they were weird. After all, I used to make gluten on purpose as part of the macrobiotic diet. He went on to tell me to avoid all forms of gluten, to check every label on every prepared food. I took his advice and stopped eating gluten immediately; or so I thought.

I didn't know at that point that eating the tiny piece of sacrament bread at church would matter. It took me six

● ● ●

weeks to get a clue, and the last time I took it I ended up in bed for three days. That week I was so horribly exhausted and in pain I could only work nine hours. The following Sunday I took my own gluten-free cracker. The result was astounding. I had no pain and worked twenty-six hours that week. So I knew for sure gluten was the problem.

The last time I ate gluten was 15 June 2012. By my sons' weddings in August and September, my weight had dropped still further and I was a 91lb skeleton. I looked dreadful and spoiled the wedding photos. In a three year period I had dropped from a clothing size 14 to a 2. All my shopping had to be done in thrift stores to keep up with the demand for new sizes. When I was a size 14, I despaired as I tried to find pants to fit properly. As I lost weight it was wonderful to be able to fit into anything again, but when I reached size 2 everything hung on me. Now I knew what it was like to be my mother.

I began to understand why she had been so emaciated and in pain every time she ate. I remember that she loved the big salads I made for her, and why she would suggest we go to a salad bar when we went shopping downtown. She tried everything to put weigh on, to no avail. She came home from work exhausted every night and just sat in her chair all evening. She died at age sixty-eight of a stomach aneurism and a brain aneurism. I am so sorry that she never found out what was wrong with her, mentally or

• • •

physically. How fortunate I feel that I have, and that I've been able to overcome it.

I had read that when you give up gluten, it takes about three months to start feeling well again. This was true for me. I also read that people, who are underweight with gluten intolerance, have a hard time putting it back on. Once I hit the three month mark, however, the weight started to come back without any problem. I made a mental goal to be 105lbs by Christmas. I reached that goal by 1 December.

In many ways I am glad that I have had bipolar disorder, diverticulosis and gluten intolerance. These illnesses have helped me understand my mother, and many other people who are suffering.

Over the years that I was eating the macrobiotic diet my mental health did not improve. My body may have been getting some extra nourishment, but it was not enough to impact my brain chemistry. Once I knew I had gluten intolerance I gave up all grains including brown rice, oats and millet. These had been my staple foods for years and I wondered then, if eating a grain based diet had actually added to my digestive problems.

I began writing this book in February 2014 and my goal was to have it ready to go to print before the end of April. However, I developed pleurisy, which I had for two months. I couldn't understand why I was so sick suddenly, and this delayed completion of the manuscript. I discovered that the problem may be related to elevation as I had moved from St George, Utah to Soda Springs, Idaho. The latter was twice as high as St George. I had to find a place in South East Idaho that was lower than Provo, where I had lived without ever having lung problems.

Moving again was a hard thing. It meant my book would have to be put on the back burner till I found the right place. I moved 31 May and within two days the pleurisy was gone. I spent from morning till night the following week cleaning and unpacking.

This meant I had to eat out a few times at a local café. The food was good, there was a nice ambience, and I enjoyed getting to know the staff. On the final day of cleaning I decided to treat myself to a chicken taco salad as I was too tired to fix anything at home. That was the last time I ate what I would call "normally."

I woke up Sunday morning still feeling full and very tired. I went into the kitchen and took a drink of water. The undigested meal came back up. I had eaten only about a third of the meal because I had become full rather quickly. I brought the rest home to finish for lunch the next day. That went straight in the bin! At first I thought I had food poisoning, but when I had water diarrhea for three days, I knew it had to be something else.

I felt an exhaustion I have never known before, an exhaustion that felt like it was in my blood. A week later, when I felt up to driving, I went into the café to ask if there

• • •

could have been any gluten in the food. Sure enough the chef had coated the chicken in flour and fried it. I had eaten maybe four little pieces of chicken, and I'm guessing I felt full quickly because the flour was stopping me digesting. I've often wondered since I was diagnosed gluten intolerant, what would happen if I ate wheat again. Now I know.

After a year of not eating gluten, I was able to eat corn again without any apparent side effects, and this spring I began eating oats again with seemingly no problem. If only I had known what I know now.

After the bout with the taco salad I went online to look up the symptoms of Celiac disease. Several people had commented that I must have the illness when I told them I couldn't eat even a crumb of bread. I had tried to ignore what they were saying as I didn't want to think about having something that sounded incurable.

As I researched I discovered that I had all the symptoms of Celiac disease. Once again I decided that I would never take a drug for it, and began to look up alternatives. This led me to what I believe is the answer and I have embraced the Specific Carbohydrate Diet. At time of writing I have been on this diet a month, and am feeling a lot better.

I have never felt that gluten-free foods were healthy, or that they were the answer to this growing problem. They seem to me to be expensive, dead foods.

• • •

This has been confirmed to me through my studies. Apparently, research and testing has been done on people who have been one to ten years gluten free. The findings are not surprising to me. In the group that was followed for ten years, only 43% recovery of the gut was noted. This is unacceptable to me. I know there has to be a way to heal this condition, and I feel, after extensive study, that the Specific Carbohydrate Diet is probably the solution.

Recently I've begun to pay more attention to what shoppers are putting in their carts at the grocery store. I have noticed that most people are buying predominantly carbohydrates; bread, cereal, pizza, crackers, pastries, beans, pasta, potatoes. I honestly believe that we have become a nation, maybe even a world, addicted to sugar.

All carbohydrates turn to sugar in the digestive process. Add the use of cane sugar, soda, and ice cream, chocolate and so on, and you have a recipe for the complete breakdown of the digestive tract.

CHAPTER FIVE

INTO THE ABYSS

At the age of thirty-four, when I met my husband, I thought my ship had come in. He seemed to be all that I had hoped and more, but his behavior towards me changed dramatically after we became engaged. I started to doubt myself and my self-worth began to plummet. When I saw myself through his eyes, I wondered why he wanted to marry me. I ascribed his behavior to pre-wedding nerves. Almost immediately after the wedding I became pregnant, and by the age of thirty-eight I had given birth to three children.

• • •

MISSION IMPROBABLE

I spent hundreds of hours as a teenager working to keep my mother's house clean. I took care of my siblings and did a variety of paid jobs after school and on Saturdays so I'd have spending money. I went to college, trained to be a school teacher and a cook, and ran several businesses. I'd traveled across the United States alone, and gained admittance to BYU on a master's program without a bachelor's degree. I considered myself pretty competent, so why now did I now feel so hopeless and worthless?

With so much experience under my belt, I thought my own home and family would be easy to manage; but that turned out not to be the case. With the birth of each child, I became increasingly stressed, exhausted and unhinged. I felt like I was living in a nightmare. I had become my husband's prisoner, with no means of escape and nowhere to go if I did.

At the time I didn't know what was happening to me, and I was made to believe that the problems were entirely mine. Thanks to my childhood training at the hands of my mother, I believed I was worthless, and his judgment of me confirmed it. With each succeeding year I was bullied, berated, criticized, and treated like an incompetent child. For those four years I slept no more than four hours a night because of the stress of living with him.

I was isolated from friends. Phone calls to my family in England were not allowed. I had to ask my husband for every penny I needed, and was required to

• • •

give an accounting of how it was spent. If I went anywhere, which was rare, I had to give a full and detailed report of where I had been and what had happened.

He was the boss, he earned and controlled the money and I was the inept underling. He had contempt and disdain for everything I did and said, and he constantly attacked my mothering of the children. I feared my husband, especially as he presented himself to friends and family as the rational one, the one that had it all together.

I began suffering extreme anxiety. I didn't know what to do. I knew something was really wrong. How could I live like this for the rest of my life? As the abuse escalated and his words became physical, I finally fell to my knees and asked God for help. My answer was to tell him to leave. I was shocked! I never would have dreamed of leaving him. It was the fall of 1994, and that evening he said he couldn't even stand being in the same room as me. I went berserk and screamed at him to get out. That night he moved back in with his parents.

During those four years I'd had no sense of what married life was really like, and felt more alone with him than when I was single. I also felt like I was a single parent because he did not want to be involved in day to day family activities. By the end of those four years I no longer knew who I was. I felt numb, and was hardly able to communicate with anyone.

● ● ●

In the early days of our separation I hoped and prayed for resolution and reconciliation, but by the time divorce court loomed, I wanted to kill myself. It wasn't the thought of losing him that terrified me; it was the thought I might have to go back to him. On the one hand I was afraid to be alone with the children, who were so young and dependent on me for everything. The alternative was to remain trapped, dominated and controlled, and to never know what my husband was going to do next.

He had threatened me repeatedly that if I divorced him, he would take the children away from me. Little did he know that his tactics on me wouldn't work with the court system. He was a big bully in our little pond, but a tin-pot dictator as far as the law was concerned.

One evening, after eighteen months of separation, I was impressed to invite him over to talk, and further impressed to ask him a series of questions. I could tell from his answers that he actually thought things were improving. My final question addressed how he would feel if his mother died. His response was "totally alone." That's when I knew there was no hope for our marriage.

My relationship with my husband's family had not been particularly close. I never felt accepted by them, especially by his mother, with whom I discovered he had a very unhealthy relationship. Marrying into his family was like jumping from the frying pan into the fire. His people had the same kind of mental and emotional problems as mine;

• • •

there were just less of them. They say if you don't resolve the childhood issues you have with your own family, you just go on and recreate them with someone else's. That's exactly what I did. I'd married my mother.

As a legal immigrant I was a permanent resident, but an alien nonetheless. I had no family support from England and none from his parents either. From the day he moved out his family never once called and asked me what happened. I guess they were satisfied with his version of things.

When I filed for divorce a few months after that interview, it was me that ended up totally alone. I had the children, but I had to share them with people who could care less about me. I almost lost my reason and could barely cope with the demands of daily living. Only the thought that my children needed a mother, prevented me from cracking up completely and taking my own life.

Over the years, even after the divorce, my husband tried to make me the scapegoat for his bad behavior. He reasoned that the problems in our marriage had been fifty-fifty, that the divorce was as much my fault. After all, I was so crazy, how could he have behaved any differently towards me? Neither he nor I could see at the time that it was his attitude and behavior towards me that sent me into a mental and emotional decline. He said I was the problem, and I thought I was. No wonder I almost ended up in a mental hospital.

• • •

MISSION IMPROBABLE

By the time I was fifty-six years old I realized I had been controlled my entire life by one person or another. Eighteen years after the divorce I came to find out that my relationship with someone I considered my best friend, was a continuation of my relationship with my husband. They say you teach people how to treat you, but unfortunately, when you have been groomed your entire life to behave a certain way and to respond to certain treatment, it's hard to make sense of what is really happening to you. No wonder we need trained therapists who can see what is going on from a neutral perspective.

I know now that divorce was my only option, but over the years I have anguished about it. I knew it would have a detrimental effect on my children, but I also knew that when a man abuses his wife, he is also abusing his children, and in the end it is a mercy for them as well. My youngest son, as a teenager, criticized me for divorcing his dad. I replied, as I wish I could have replied years before, to the silent judgments and criticisms of my so-called friends and neighbors:

"Why would a woman, at the age of forty, living in a basement apartment, with no extended family support, no money, and no hope of being able to work to adequately support her children, leave her only provider?"

After the initial relief of getting away from my husband and starting, what I hoped, would be a new life, I went into another downward spiral. I was upset and

• • •

anxious most of the time. I never knew how I was going to feel when I woke up in the morning. I could be energetic on the one hand and a few weeks later I would run out of steam completely.

After the divorce I agreed to one-on-one counseling, then medication for depression. By that time I had been divorced two years, I was on food stamps and HUD housing. I found taking handouts from the government demoralizing in the extreme. I'd emigrated from England with high hopes of living the American dream, of living in a society free of socialism and council housing and the dole. I never imagined for a second that I would end up as a welfare recipient as the mother of three children. It has been said that it is not being poor that is the problem, it's what poverty does to you. I felt degraded, embarrassed and stigmatized, which added further stress to my already traumatic existence.

My husband's hatred and harassment grew after the divorce, as did my fear of him. He kept threatening to take the children away from me, and after one particularly vicious phone conversation, I called a friend for help. He told me I needed to get away, far away, from him, and never look back. I broke down sobbing, and knew he was right.

I didn't drive in England. I was actually afraid to learn, as I think my non-driver, bipolar mother must have been. It was not until after the separation from my husband

• • •

that I plucked up the courage to take lessons. I was assured by my driving instructor that I would gain a new lease on life, and that I would love the freedom that would come with it. I was thirty-nine years old and he was right. It would be another six years until I finally drove away from my husband for good.

One day I asked my therapist what he thought about my desire to move away. I wanted to know if it was morally wrong for me to take the children away from their father. I was shocked at his reply. He asked me what I wanted! I avoided answering and went into a speech about how a mother's job was to nurture and protect her children, and that I feared what my ex-husband was capable of. I feared that his violence would escalate and that he might kill me. The therapist again asked me what I wanted, and I broke down in tears and said I wanted to get as far away from him as possible, that I could no longer take the stress of what he was saying, threatening and doing to me.

The reason I was shocked by his question was because I had spent my life trying to make everything work. I had given my ex-husband liberal visitation of the children, and even asked him at one point if he wanted to see the children every day. He said no.

I took the blame for all the problems, in my family of origin and then in my marriage. I had to fix them because they were my fault. I tried to take care of everyone else's feelings, but neglected my own. The truth is I had been given and had accepted the lifetime role of scapegoat.

I tried not to feel the awfulness of the situation, but I had to admit to myself and to my therapist, that I dreamed of a life where I no longer had to interact with my children's father. In fact, I used to wish that I had been widowed, because I wouldn't have him to deal with anymore. I might even get some sympathy and support, instead of judgment and criticism from the people around me.

Marriage and motherhood had been, for me, a lifelong desire. I never wanted to work outside the home. I wanted to create a happy family, a secure, warm home. I never had any desire for a career. Try as I might, I could not seem to do what needed to be done to create the family I yearned for. I thought, however naively, that I could have a happy family, and that my life could turn out.

Five years after the divorce, a move away seemed the only way to find peace and healing in my own life. Divorce had not ended the abuse and harassment, and it was with great trepidation that I decided to sell everything and move to Oregon. Everything we owned was either in the trunk of the car or left in a small storage unit.

When we moved out of state, my children were seven, eight and ten-years-old. My poor daughter had a broken growth plate in her leg and was on crutches; all three children had broken hearts, along with my own. What a piteous sight we must have looked to the policemen who

● ● ●

cautioned me for speeding on a distant country road, in my anxiety to get us somewhere safe, fast.

Little did I know then, that this move was really the beginning of the end of life as we knew it. The increased stress of moving to a place where we knew nobody, with very little money and no job, took its toll. My home-based business would prove to be unsuccessful in our new location, and in time, along with several other factors, I was propelled into my second major depressive episode.

My new doctor prescribed yet another anti-depressant. On this drug my mania increased and the ups and downs of my moods became alarmingly close together. Eventually I became completely dysfunctional and could not leave the house except under cover of darkness, and that was only to put out the trash.

I was nervous, moody and upset, and although I tried my best to appear normal to neighbors and friends, and especially to my children, I felt as though I was careening downward into a terrible hell. My behavior became increasingly erratic and unpredictable. Stress and anxiety became full-blown panic attacks. I also developed lung trouble, a side-effect of the anti-depressant, and had to manage the problem by taking large doses of Vitamin E to help me breathe.

Medford, Oregon, had a pretty sluggish economy with few jobs, so I decided after two and a half years to move to Portland. I hoped I would have better success with

• • •

my business. I sold my car to someone I knew in Provo, Utah, so that I could afford to make the move, hoping the money I got for it would be enough to sustain us for a few months until I got on my feet again.

It was fall when I left my children with friends in Medford and made the twelve hour drive alone to Provo. At this point, my mania was at the worst it had ever been. I look back in horror as I recall the journey. I drove without stopping, with the car window rolled down, singing all the way, at the top of my lungs!

When I arrived in Provo I was super excitable, and I heard later that the woman I'd delivered the car to, said she preferred me depressed. I returned to Medford a day later with friends who were going home, then packed the U-Haul and drove it to Portland.

The mania was mistaken by my new church friends as love. I was gushing with love and became popular overnight. Then came the crash and, not surprisingly, everyone turned away from me. As the days shortened and became colder and the holidays loomed, I went spiraling down into the worst depression of my life, my third and final episode.

The usual distractions like reading and movies didn't help to take away the dreadful feelings that robbed me of my peace of mind. I felt like I was in a deep, dark pit with no way out. My actions were slowed down and I just wanted to bury myself in a shroud and go to sleep forever.

• • •

MISSION IMPROBABLE

Things that I thought were real were not. I couldn't make decisions because I wasn't sure what was best. I would mull things over in my mind constantly and my thoughts raced until I wanted to scream for them to stop. It was literally like being a prisoner in my own mind.

All was chaos, instability and despair. I felt at the mercy of my own thoughts and delusions. People were scary and unpredictable and I felt that I was at everyone's mercy. Life had no meaning as I tried to make it through each day.

I suffered extreme bouts of self-hate and self-loathing. I believed everything negative anyone said about me. I believed I was just a worthless problem. I really wanted to cease to exist. I literally felt that there was nothing left for me. I wanted to die and get it over with. I couldn't get up any more. I was completely and utterly spent.

Clinical depression is frightening. Mental and emotional anguish is accompanied by physical pain. My whole body felt tortured. Nothing helped me feel better, including therapy. I could hardly stand to be touched. No matter how many times I was told people cared, or that things would get better, I never believed it.

I used to feel like I was born into a basement, and as the years of my life went by I could never get above the ground floor. I was always looking for something or

● ● ●

someone to come along and make it better, but it never happened.

I had been well educated, traveled, run my own businesses, been married, had children, and was capable in so many ways; yet I felt inexperienced and under-developed. It was like being a child in an adult body, and although I had always been very competent, I felt increasingly unable to run my own life.

I had become unstable mentally, emotionally, socially, physically and financially. I felt rootless and was always living on the edge. Other people grew and progressed while I continued waiting for my life to start.

I could no longer work and the thought of just picking up the phone to try to get work filled me with dread. I could barely keep the house going or teach my children. By Christmas I could barely function and in January, though I couldn't even stand to leave the house, I went to the library to research bipolar disorder. It took me all my strength to go.

● ● ●

MISSION IMPROBABLE

• • •

CHAPTER SIX

TRUEHOPE: DEBBIE STEPHAN'S LEGACY

That trip to the library saved my life.

I had been a research assistant for a year as a graduate student and I knew how to find things in popular journals. I typed the words "bipolar disorder" into the search field of the computer. Nothing came up. Then I typed "manic depression" and up came dozens of articles.

I scanned them for symptoms listed and went into shock, realizing that I had many of them. As the awful truth

● ● ●

sank in, I started to develop a migraine, and had to go home.

I managed to copy about fifteen articles, most of them a page or so long. All I wanted was to find out what the symptoms of bipolar disorder were, and whether they matched mine. The next day, while lying down recovering from the exhaustion that accompanies migraine headaches, I read the short articles, leaving the longest until last.

As I read the first fourteen, I became increasingly alarmed. I realized that the case histories recounted described people who were being medicated, but were not functioning. I knew right then, that there was no way I was going on medication. I knew I would never get the help and healing I needed from taking more psychotropic drugs.

Looking back at the condition I was in, I see that I would have eventually lost my mind and my freedom completely, and would have been locked up in a mental hospital with no hope of ever getting out.

I picked up the final article which was titled "Bipolar Breakthrough"-seven pages of information that would literally change my life forever. It described how a Canadian woman named Debbie Stephan, after years of suffering, had committed suicide leaving ten children. Her husband, Tony, had done everything in his power to help her, to no avail. He felt overwhelmed by her illness and then by her tragic death.

• • •

One of the children, Joseph, who was in the throes of puberty when his mother died, became increasingly troubled and violent. Tony feared for his son's safety, as well as for the safety of the entire family, and continued to look for answers. One day while at work, he met a man named David Hardy. The ensuing conversation between the two men would change the lives of the Stephan family, and subsequently, the lives of thousands of mentally ill people.

David, a biologist, went on to tell Tony about his work as an animal feed specialist, and specifically about a supplement he had created for the pig industry. Tail-biting syndrome, a sometimes lethal behavior in pigs, was a huge problem. The animals could become extremely aggressive, maiming each other as they went into violent frenzies. After much research and study, David came to the conclusion that pigs, which are omnivorous and will eat anything, were not getting complete nutrition. The result was a chemical imbalance in their brains, which could only be alleviated by introducing a specific blend of minerals, vitamins and amino acids into their diets.

David concluded this first conversation with Tony by saying that if it could be done for pigs, it could be done for people. Thus a close working relationship was formed as the two men labored to produce a micronutrient composition that would address Joseph's condition.

● ● ●

By the age of fifteen Tony's son was on the verge of permanent and secure hospitalization. Although the supplement was nowhere near ready, and was not yet in capsule form, he was introduced to the concoction by teaspoon. Regular doses at intervals throughout each day led to incredible results. Within a month his mood swings had stopped, and Joseph's sanity was saved. The micronutrients, which when encapsulated were bottled and labeled EMPowerplus, would keep him out of mental hospitals permanently.

His older sister, Autumn, had also exhibited symptoms of bipolar disorder throughout her teens. She married and had a baby boy, but after the birth of her son she went into full-blown psychosis. She was in and out of psychiatric hospitals for three years, and her marriage was on the verge of collapse. Increasingly unable to take care of her little son, she was advised against having any more children.

Tony's daughter was resistant to taking the micronutrients and in desperation her father made her take them. Gradually her symptoms subsided and Autumn recovered completely. She has been symptom free for over seventeen years and now has four children.

Autumn has written a book The Promise of Hope which documents her mother's descent into mental illness and tragic suicide, her own terrible nightmare with bipolar disorder, and her valiant recovery. She now lives a very

• • •

happy and productive life as a wife and mother, public speaker, political advocate for the mentally ill, and promoter of the EMPowerplus. Autumn also has an online blog discussing various aspects of mental illness and recovery.

Tony Stephan and David Hardy worked together for twenty years to build the non-profit organization they named Truehope Nutritional Support Ltd. In the process, over a hundred thousand adults and children in one hundred countries have resolved serious mental illness. It has been discovered that the micronutrients not only address the symptoms of bipolar disorder, but also a range of other illnesses of the central nervous system.

This may sound like a simplistic solution, but I agree with Tony Stephan who said that someday mental illness is going to be seen as nothing more than a nutritional deficiency. Nevertheless, out of small and simple things, great things can and do come to pass. This is one of them.

Truehope has developed a website where research has been documented, success stories have been told, and information has been collected for the educating of those who are desperately seeking answers. The website and phone information for Truehope, is listed at the end of this book. I urge anyone who is suffering with any form of mental illness, or who is a caregiver or relative of someone who is ill, to go on the websites and study what has been and is being done by Truehope, and then to call

● ● ●

them and discuss with a counselor the best way to proceed.

Although the EMPowerplus was created to address serious disorders of the central nervous system, the general population is also getting relief from stress and finding renewed ability to focus.

I believe that Anthony Stephan and David Hardy are pioneers in the field of micro nutrition as it relates to mental illness, and if anyone should be awarded the Nobel Peace Prize, it is these two men.

CHAPTER SEVEN

ONE DAY AT A TIME

After I read "Bipolar Breakthrough" I called Truehope and asked for further information. I told them my situation and asked if there was any way I could get help. The counselor, told me to write a letter to them detailing my mental health history, and describing my current situation.

She told me there was a program in place called the Perpetual Health Fund which could assist people with part of the cost of the EMPowerplus. This fund has been established because so many people with mental illness cannot work, and are on disability and welfare. Truehope is a non-profit organization. Their main focus is getting people

• • •

well, so they do everything they can to help people with the cost.

I wrote a long letter and sent it off to Canada. Within a couple of weeks I received a phone call from Tony Stephan himself. He informed me that I had been selected to receive EMPowerplus at no cost, and that I would need to communicate with the Truehope wellness team on a regular basis. I thanked him profusely, hung up the phone and burst into tears. At last I was going to get help!

I spoke to a wellness counselor that day who said I would have to fill out symptom evaluation forms for two weeks, and send them in to their office. The information would be logged into a computer as a record for future monitoring and evaluation. I was required to fill in these forms every day, and mail them in each week. Eventually I was able to buy a computer and could fill them in online. These would be viewed by Truehope staff, and I could access them with a username and password. They were available to me in graph and chart form so that I could see my progress. This information is still available today, and I have been able to use it to show people how my condition changed over time.

As Truehope has become better known over the past decade, many more people are calling in for help. Truehope wants everyone who calls to be able to get the nutrients-at a reduced price when necessary-although the EMPowerplus can no longer be offered for free. Their

• • •

reasoning is that if everyone pays something, many more others can get help, until they are able to afford to pay the full price. To get on the wellness fund, potential participants must send in proof of income from the previous year's tax forms.

I decided to keep a journal describing in detail how I was able to get off medication and on to the micronutrients. I continued to keep the journal until I was able to return to work. The following information comes from two spiral bound notebooks in which I kept a daily log of my progress.

It should be noted that in the seven years I was on psychotropic medication I tried around four or five different kinds, and never took them simultaneously. There were also long periods when I was not on any medication, mainly because they were not really working, and the terrible side effects made a normal life impossible.

In preparation to start the program, I was told by Truehope staff to cut my anti-depressant down, from 30mg to 25mg, one week before I started on the micronutrient regimen. It was around noon on 12 February 2003, when the UPS man knocked on the door holding my first package containing two bottles of EMPowerplus. I immediately called my Truehope counselor for instructions.

She told me to take one capsule immediately with lunch, then two more with a mid-afternoon snack. I followed her instructions and noticed that I felt a little "spaced out"

● ● ●

for the rest of the day. I had a minor stomach upset in the evening and went to bed at 11:45pm. I fell asleep within fifteen minutes, which was unusual for me, because it often took me over an hour to get to sleep.

I slept till 5:00am, when I had to get up to use the bathroom, and fell right back to sleep till 6:30am. When I awoke that day I felt a calm I had never felt before in my life! All day the calm persisted, which was also unusual because I always felt very anxious. My head was clear and my thoughts were orderly. My speech was slower and the angry edge to my voice had softened. I also felt more positive. That day, 13 February, I took two capsules after each meal, the last being around 4:30pm. That made a total of six.

That night I started getting tired around 9:00pm, but wanted some time alone after my children had gone to bed. I watched some TV until about 10:45pm and had to go to bed because I couldn't stay awake. It took me only a few minutes to fall asleep and I slept deeply, without dreaming, until 6:30am.

I am including these details about my sleep patterns because sleep deprivation created high stress for me after I had my children. The abuse in my marriage compounded the problem, and over a fifteen year period my stress became a chronic and debilitating condition.

Getting to bed early was usually very difficult, because it took me hours to fall asleep. As soon as I lay

• • •

down my brain would go into overdrive, and my thoughts would race. I would dread going to bed. I could fall asleep in front of the TV by 10:00pm, but just getting into bed meant I would lie there tossing and turning. I also had a terrible time sleeping through the night, and tended to wake up early. In fact, no matter how late I went to bed, I could never sleep in. By the time I was in my mid-forties, I often stayed up till 2:00am. I couldn't understand it; especially as all my life I liked to go to bed early and had been an early riser. Being able to finally get to sleep at a decent time was wonderful.

I noticed the second day on EMPowerplus I was even more calm and clear headed. I didn't feel so on edge and was a lot more relaxed. I also noticed that the pain and stiffness in my neck and shoulders had decreased, along with the pain in my lower back.

Day three was Valentine's Day and I was instructed by my counselor to increase the capsules to nine. Unfortunately, I forgot the last dose after dinner and took it at 8:00pm, resulting in an upsurge in brain energy. It was after midnight when I finally fell asleep, but this showed me clearly why I needed to take all the capsules by 6:00pm. Subsequently, I tried to take them no later than 3:00pm, especially as my goal was to be in bed by 9:00pm. That day I awoke at 5:30am and noticed an all-round energy increase, although I had to take a two hour nap in the afternoon to make up for the short night's sleep.

• • •

MISSION IMPROBABLE

Saturday, day four, I was positive and felt happier. I still didn't feel all that sociable, but I made myself go to the bank and to the church Valentine's party in the evening. I ate dinner and left early because I didn't feel very comfortable socially. This new experience in healing my brain made me extra nervous around people. I was so involved in the process, watching myself and my body to see how I was thinking, feeling and acting, that being around people made me on edge.

I had been told the day before to cut my medication to 20mg and on that fourth day took twelve EMPowerplus capsules, four after each meal. I did so by 4:00pm and was really tired by 10:00pm, but stayed up until 11:00pm. Bad habits can be hard to break!

I had a very strange night waking up every two hours and had the weirdest dreams. I'm not actually sure that I was dreaming because I just kept seeing strange shapes and colors before my eyes, like luminous DNA strands all joined together.

16 February found me feeling good and positive, but very tired because of the disturbed night. I was still a little irritable and my head felt tight across the forehead, and across the back of my neck, which was stiff again.

I took fifteen capsules, five with each meal, by 5:00pm, and began noticing some constipation. I also had a low grade headache during the afternoon.

● ● ●

S. Deborah Fryer

Monday 17 February came and I felt anxious and nervous about going to the full loading dose of eighteen capsules. I became calmer as the day progressed and spent my time quietly resting and doing some sewing.

I went to bed at 10:00pm and was asleep within a half hour, but had another restless night filled with graphic and violent dreams. I got up to go to the bathroom and my head and neck felt very tight and stiff. My lungs felt constricted and my breathing was labored. This was a sure sign to me that the medication I had taken was beginning to be cleansed from my body.

The following day, Tuesday 18 February, found me much more energetic after seven and a half hours' sleep. I did chores and sewed for some time. I was fairly focused but didn't feel like doing any mental work, like reading or writing. I was still feeling unsociable and irritable and could barely talk, even to my children. I had eighteen capsules split into three doses and was counseled to take the 20mg of the anti-depressant, this time right before bed.

Day eight found me somewhat depressed on waking and I had to make myself get up, shower and run errands. I did some sewing, but would rather have watched TV. I had a hard time focusing and had to force myself to fill in the symptom forms and write in my Truehope notebook. I felt irritable and sad, and had a disturbed night, sleeping a total of seven and a half hours.

MISSION IMPROBABLE

    Thursday, 20 February found me extremely tired and I didn't want to do anything. I had an appointment with a new therapist, but didn't feel well enough to drive, so I asked a friend to take me. By lunchtime I was even more depressed and got very angry with my children, which was upsetting to us all. The exhaustion and depression intensified, so I called Truehope who told me to decrease the medication to 15mg at bedtime. By dinnertime I was weepy and didn't want to talk, think or do anything.

    The next morning I awoke feeling happy. I had slept nine hours with a bathroom visit at 5:00am. At 11:30am I suddenly felt very tired, and an hour later developed a headache and nausea. My mind was clear, but the headache, which bordered on a migraine, was draining. I also had loose bowels and felt pretty upset and irritable. I was worried about what was happening to me, and didn't want to interact with anyone. I had to force myself to run a couple of errands, and finally took some ibuprofen and went to bed at 10:00pm.

    Day eleven started with me feeling exhausted and worn out with the headache from the day before. I planned to finish my sewing project but was too tired. I had to run some errands but didn't really feel up to it. I didn't take my first six capsules of EMPowerplus till lunchtime, and within an hour had another headache. By 5:00pm I had taken all eighteen, and had to take more headache medicine.

• • •

It should be noted here that as a rule I never took any form of pain medicine, or any other drugs for that matter, even when I had migraines. I usually just let them run their course, but with all the other symptoms I was having, I needed some relief. A few times, when I have had a urinary tract infection, I had to take an antibiotic, but I didn't like taking them and only did so when there was no alternative.

I suddenly became very tired and developed flu-like symptoms, although my mind was still clear. I read a few pages of a book, but my eyes began to hurt and I had to stop. I didn't feel depressed, but was concerned enough to call Truehope, and left a message.

Sunday 23 February dawned. I felt better, more at peace, but still very tired. My neck was stiff and painful on the left side, but I had no headache. I really didn't want to see anyone, so I stayed home instead of going to church, and rested.

The next day I was depressed and short-tempered. I cut the medication down to 10mg that night and felt much better the next morning.

Day fourteen arrived and I felt happier, more positive and didn't mind being around people. I'd made it two whole weeks on the wellness program! I called Truehope and was told to cut back to twelve capsules as the bad headaches and depression was a sure sign that the psychotropic medications were cleansing from my system.

I discovered during those early days that the body really does dictate our needs, and when I was putting off taking the EMPowerplus until lunchtime, my brain was telling me it was too much. The Truehope counselor confirmed that I had done the right thing.

On day fifteen I had an active morning. I was positive, happy and sociable, but became very tired during the afternoon and had to take a long nap, even though I had slept nine hours the night before. I woke from my nap sad and depressed and called Truehope for advice.

I was told to cut the medication to 5mg and increase the EMPowerplus to fourteen capsules. I was becoming very nervous at this point because I had been told by Truehope that the drug I was taking was highly addictive. I was worried about what might happen next.

The next day I felt much better, although still tired. However, my body felt stronger and my mind was clearer and more focused. I felt good, calm and fairly positive, and that night I slept nine hours.

The following day, day seventeen, I felt well and relaxed but still a little tired. My mind was clear, but I wasn't up to any kind of mental exertion. I did a few minutes' reading and later that day had to attend a meeting in the evening. I was cautious about socializing because I felt awkward and nervous. Before I left home I forgot to take

• • •

my last four capsules of EMPowerplus, so I took only ten capsules that day.

1 March was a roller coaster of emotion. I felt happy in the morning and became increasingly irritable and upset by evening. 9:00pm found me very depressed, and I wondered if that meant it was time to stop taking the anti-depressant completely. I slept only six hours that night, but felt better when I woke up. I took no more medication Sunday, and on Monday morning called Truehope to tell them what I had done. They agreed that I had done the right thing, and told me to increase the EMPowerplus to sixteen capsules. So it was that in nineteen days I was completely off medication. I was shocked at how fast this had happened.

I have included this detailed daily description of my early days on the wellness program so that anyone contemplating getting off medication, in favor of the micronutrients, can see what is involved, and that it can be done. It is not easy, and everyone's experience will be different, but mine confirmed to me that what Truehope told me about the process was accurate. I also learned how important it was to call my Truehope counselor so I could be well monitored, and that no problem was too small for her to address and discuss.

I also want professionals in the field of medicine, psychiatry and psychology who may read this book, to see that my reduction and eventual dispensing with medications

• • •

was done under close supervision. I am concerned that the medical profession also understands that Truehope is a responsible entity, with eighteen years of experience in helping people to transfer from drug therapy to brain nutrition. It may be argued that the supervision was not medical, but I had no doctor or medical insurance, and had to rely solely on the support staff at Truehope, whose guidance proved excellent in every instance.

Each day I filled in the symptom evaluation forms religiously, and sent them in weekly to Truehope. When my forms were received they were entered into a computer program which recorded and graphed my symptoms, sleep patterns, and the amount of EMPowerplus and medication I consumed. I can still view these charts today, and have shown them to many people. Over the following months I continued to keep a daily record of my progress, and I have them in my possession today. They are available for anyone to examine them.

The next four months from March through the end of June were difficult in the extreme. The whole process should probably have been undertaken in a sanatorium of some kind. However, because I was poor, and had no kind of health insurance, I had no choice but to take care of myself. Many people have gone through this process without medical support, and have been successful. Supervision by a doctor is recommended by Truehope and is, of course, preferable.

• • •

I ended up housebound and bed-ridden for three months. In my case, the protracted withdrawals from these psychotropic drugs were akin to a really bad flu. It was a terrible ordeal. I suffered from increased anxiety, panic, depression, diarrhea, body aches, nerve pains in my arms and shoulders, headaches, nausea, fatigue, lethargy, insomnia and suicidal ideation. On two occasions I had to call Truehope to help me through the worst of the suicidal thoughts and feelings of deep despair.

I must emphasize at this point, that the drug withdrawals were the cause of my dysfunction at this point, not the EMPowerplus. Withdrawals will happen, whether someone is on the EMPowerplus or not. They can be nasty; and certain drugs have worse side-effects than others, as well as worse withdrawals than others. The effects can be debilitating, there is no way to say it less alarmingly. However, I am living proof that they can be negotiated and overcome. I would suffer them all over again to get to where I am today.

My children spent the majority of that summer with their father. I was glad they didn't have to see me going through the whole of this terrible process. The months went by in a blur, but by the time June came, I felt a lot better, though still rather weak. However, I determined to get myself out of bed and get moving, and gradually I was able to build up my strength through walking and chores. There were times during those months when I couldn't even walk

● ● ●

across my living room, but soon I could walk around our apartment building, and then around the complex. It took great determination to pull myself up and get back into life.

Bipolar disorder made me very hostile because often I didn't know what was real, what and who to trust or how to make decisions. Fear of the unknown made me incapable of knowing how to proceed in many areas of life. Years of illness led to a kind of defensiveness that sabotaged the efforts of others to be helpful. I had a hard time asking for help, as I didn't like appearing vulnerable. I had to trust Truehope and what my counselor was telling me. I didn't know the end from the beginning, but I did feel that there was hope to be well in the future using this remedy. Drugs had made my condition worse, so I had to do something different.

As a potential program participant, I recognized and appreciated that it was my Truehope counselor's job to obtain as much information as possible from me. Details of medicines I had taken, past and present, were of paramount importance if the journey from drug therapy to micro-nutrition was going to be smooth and as uneventful as possible. I never found the questions into my medical history invasive, and in my experience, the more a counselor knew about my background, the better they were able to assist and advise me.

The staff at Truehope was professional, caring and committed to the cause of mental wellness. They

• • •

rejoiced with me when they saw me conquering my disease. My counselor spent hours and hours helping me to understand what was happening in my body and my mind, and was a wonderful cheer leader. I shall ever be grateful for her experienced and skilled counseling.

MISSION IMPROBABLE

CHAPTER EIGHT

OUT OF DARKNESS

In March 2003, after a month or more on the Truehope program, I climbed out of my bed, terribly sick from drug withdrawals, and prayed for a miracle. In my debilitated condition, I knew God was the only one I could turn to. I knew from past experience that He would help me. I was living in a new city and didn't know many people. I had done everything I could to support my family, but I had no idea how I would manage financially as I walked this road to wellness. I didn't know how long the road would be, but I had to take it. I had no idea how I was going to survive financially, how I would get through the months ahead.

● ● ●

Within days of that prayer I got a phone call from my sister in England telling me dad wanted to send me some money. I was shocked because I had no relationship with him, or with anyone in my family. It was hard for me to accept money from him because, when I had seen him five years earlier, he made it clear to me that he wanted nothing to do with me. It didn't make sense that he wanted to send me money, but I accepted it as God's solution to my predicament, and gave my bank account information to my sister. The money that was deposited turned out to be exactly what I needed sustain us until I felt well enough to go back to work. These were the worst of times, but they turned out to also be the best of times, because I was on my way to having a life.

I didn't feel completely well in July when I decided to get out of bed and go find a job. I felt like a newborn lamb, unsteady on my feet, not knowing what I would be like around people or in a job situation. I had been self-employed most of my adult life, because I found working away from home, and working for other people, too stressful.

Having no car, I focused my efforts on getting a job at the strip mall fifteen minutes' walk from our apartment complex. I knew if I could work there, the daily walk would do me good, and I wouldn't be too far away from home. It took me a couple of weeks to secure the position as clerk at the GNC store. One day when I called

• • •

in, the owner was there, and after talking to me for fifteen minutes, offered me the job on the spot.

I started work on 17 July doing thirty hours a week at minimum wage. I had been on EMPowerplus for just over five months. I was worried about whether I could learn all that I had to learn about the products, and how to work the cash register, among other things. However, I soon got the hang of things, and even had a good rapport with the young girl who worked the overlapping shift.

The owner soon developed confidence in me as I cleaned and organized the store from top to bottom so it functioned better. I also cleared out the storeroom, which was full of old signs and boxes. I offered to create a filing system to house seven years of payroll for all the three stores the boss owned. Working at this job showed me that I was really getting better; my stamina was improving and I could focus again. I worked through the end of April 2004, and only gave notice when the owner told me the store was not running at a profit, and that he would probably have to close.

I had been on the EMPowerplus a year and three months by this time and felt strong enough to make the move back to Utah, where I heard the building industry was booming. I felt confident I could build a business detailing new houses for building contractors. So, once again, I packed up my little family and moved yet again.

● ● ●

It was a stressful move. I was a nervous long-distance driver, and this was the furthest I had ever driven. I was forced to break the journey into four days in order to survive it. Mother's day weekend 2004, we pulled into St George in our little U-Haul truck. I realize now that this was a huge undertaking for someone in my condition. Recovering from bipolar disorder takes time, and with the complications of intermittent, ongoing drug withdrawals, a trip like that was overwhelming.

Although it was hard adapting to the hot desert climate, it was nice to be in a warmer and sunnier place. That summer was the hottest I ever knew in St George. On 4 July it was 117 degrees! I could hardly stand to be outside, even at night.

Throughout my life I had been good at cleaning and organizing, and always enjoyed making a house into a home. So Mission Impeccable: Turning Houses into Homes was born, and while the work was challenging in the extreme, and there were days when I wondered what I was doing, I felt at last that I was making headway towards becoming independent again. I was in my fifties, recovering from a mental illness and struggling to raise teenagers. Some days I had to pray for additional strength just to be able to carry on.

Before being on the wellness program with Truehope I couldn't even pick up the phone to ask women to hold skin care classes. After eighteen months on

• • •

EMPowerplus, I was approaching men on building sites to talk to them about my cleaning services.

When I began this new venture, the average house size was around fifteen hundred square feet. Over the next few years builders became more and more determined to create grander, more opulent styles. House sizes increased to as much as ten thousand square feet. At first I found them overwhelming, but in time they became routine. My physical strength grew and I was amazed at how, a few years before, I had not been able to walk around my apartment building, work or communicate with anyone.

As I built my business, I gained a reputation for being one of the few sub-contractors who showed up to work on time and when I said I would. I also became known as a detailer, someone who finished the job I started, and did it to Parade of Homes standard. I guaranteed that new home owners would not have to clean when they moved in. It was grueling work, and there were days when I came home totally exhausted, but the hard labor helped me get stronger, and the detailing helped me regain focus.

Sometimes I had to hire a crew from the local college or labor office, especially when new owners had to move into their house by a certain date. I generally hired four or five people to help me get it done in a few days. It was fun working with them, training them to do detailed cleaning. I felt that I was a good boss, and was usually respected by those I hired. This was more proof to me that I was healing, and that I could work under pressure with unskilled people, and maintain a good rapport with them.

It wasn't long before the building industry in St George collapsed. I saw the signs as early as 2006, and like many other business people, I had to diversify in order to stay afloat. I started taking care of private homes year round for people who lived there only during the winter, and did professional organizing, work that required serious focus. Later I also did some elderly care to subsidize our income.

The hard physical labor, coupled with extremes of temperature, meant that I continued to battle drug withdrawals. There were many days when I managed to go to work, but could do nothing else. Unfortunately my children paid the price as I had little energy for activities with them. I would often come home and just lie on the couch, numb from exhaustion. Meals had to be simplified, and I watched a lot of TV to try to relax and unwind.

Gradually, we settled into a routine, and life became more stable and predictable. I was earning more money than I had ever earned, and for the first time was able to take care of my family myself. Our income was still low, and there were no luxuries or vacations, but we had a roof over our heads, food on the table and the bills were paid. That, in itself, I considered a triumph.

• • •

CHAPTER NINE

NOBODY CAN TAKE CARE OF YOU LIKE YOU CAN

By the time I found Truehope I was suicidal and upset, anxious and depressed, and saw no way of ever improving my life. Many people, including well-meaning friends and therapists, tried to give me counsel about doing things to help myself feel better, but each time they did I felt as though I was being asked to climb Mount Everest. Often I was overwhelmed when any demands or expectations were made of me. It was not until I started taking the EMPowerplus that I could even think of doing the things they recommended.

Bipolar disorder, like other mental illnesses, is a chemical imbalance in the brain which affects the will. A

• • •

behavioral approach to wellness doesn't work. I never found insight therapy very helpful in connection with depression either. My brain chemistry had to first be balanced, then my thinking and behaviors could be changed or modified.

It is hard for friends and family to see someone going through an illness like this. It is frustrating when they see the sufferer can't do the things they consider normal, even easy. There is a tendency to treat the person with bipolar disorder as though they are lazy or incompetent in some way, and to attack their character when they cannot perform well or make good choices.

Someday, in the future, people will come to understand that mental illness is not a character disorder- that it is actually nothing more than a nutritional deficiency.

Before I found Truehope, there were days when I needed all my strength to shower and dress, to keep the house in order, make meals and work to support my children. When I was in a deep depression, I had no desire to do anything. As soon as I started taking EMPowerplus I began to feel better; but improvement and then healing came gradually. There have been many ups and downs on the road to wellness, and I continue to learn how to take care of myself better, and how to maximize the effects of the micronutrients.

It took me forty-nine years to become as sick as I was, so I knew it was going to take time for me to get well. I

● ● ●

was on the full loading dose of eighteen capsules (then fifteen capsules after reformulation) for bipolar disorder for six years. At that point I was able to decrease the dosage until I was finally on four capsules a day. This did not come about arbitrarily. I had often wondered when the day would arrive that I would be well enough to take the maintenance dose. It came in a way I least expected.

I had moved house and had a lot of stressful things happening close together. I suddenly started being very angry and even threw a few tantrums. I thought the stress in my life was indicating that I needed to take more. I called my counselor to discuss the problem, and we agreed that I should increase the daily intake of EMPowerplus, and I ended up taking twenty for a few days. This led to further upsets and angry tirades. Then I decided to try taking less. As soon as I decreased the capsules to twelve a day, I felt some relief. Over the next week or so I took one capsule less each day. By the time I reached four a day I felt much better.

This experience showed me that we can make errors of judgment about the amount of EMPowerplus we should take. Maintaining on four a day meant that my brain was now healed, and that I was on the way to a full recovery.

Today the EMPowerplus has been reformulated further so that the full loading dose for bipolar disorder is eight capsules. It is now renamed EMPowerplus Advanced.

• • •

There are many factors which can limit the effectiveness of the micronutrients, so it is important to do everything possible to make changes that will help EMPowerplus do its job. The following is an alphabetically ordered list of things I did to help myself through the recovery process:

ANTIBIOTICS

Antibiotics have an adverse effect on the intestines, killing good bacteria along with the bad, and interfering with the absorption of nutrients. I have rarely used them as an adult, and have tried to conquer any infection with natural antibiotics such as oil of oregano. Since I started on the EMPowerplus regimen I have had prescription antibiotics only twice for serious bladder and kidney infections. After each round I ate yogurt and fermented vegetables like sauerkraut, as well as pro-biotic supplements for about a month. This helped restore the intestinal flora in my gut.

ANXIETY

Acute anxiety often accompanied the withdrawals and so I took phosphatidyl choline, a natural anti-anxiety supplement. I ordered it from Truehope, but sometimes, when my supply ran out and I needed it quickly, I bought it from the local natural foods store.

● ● ●

CAFFEINE

I haven't had any serious caffeinated drinks since I was in my mid-twenties when I adopted a natural foods lifestyle. On one occasion, before I discovered I was bipolar, I drank a small bottle of caffeinated soda to help me stay awake when I had to drive several hundred miles in one day. The consequence was a very bad headache bordering on a migraine the next day, so I never drank anything with caffeine in it again. I don't drink tea or coffee, and have not for over thirty-two years.

DIARRHEA

In the beginning I had a few days of diarrhea caused by the antidepressants being discharged from my system. My Truehope counselor told me to chew several of Truehope's BMD calcium tablets as many times as needed to improve bowel function. This brand, which has been formulated to work with the EMPowerplus, is the only calcium which can be used.

DIET

As soon as I could get complete control of my diet when I was a college student, I began eating more whole, fresh foods. I felt happier with less meat and salt and introduced a broader array of vegetables.

● ● ●

As a child dairy and chocolate were big comfort foods for me. I drank a lot of ice-cold milk and loved cheese. However, when I was twenty-one I had three severe bouts of flu in three months. A friend suggested I give up milk as doing so had freed him of colds and other upper respiratory problems. I decided to give it a try and began to feel much better. I never drank milk again, and now cannot imagine doing so. Once I found Truehope I heard that milk can be a major cause of irritable bowel syndrome, which can have a negative effect on absorption of minerals.

I have noticed throughout my life, that eating regular meals helps me feel better. There were times when eating seemed like a chore. Eventually I came to see that eating three meals a day, as well as getting enough calories, contributes towards better sleep patterns.

I have come to the conclusion that if we are to be healthy, we need foods which contain minerals, vitamins and amino acids. I honestly believe that obesity and the proliferation of so many fad diets, has come about because the basic western diet has not been providing the nutrients we need.

DRUG WITHDRAWALS

Psychotropic medications are stored in the body's organs, fat and tissue, for up to ten years after they were last taken. As time goes by they are discharged from the

● ● ●

body. However, hot weather, hot baths and hot tubs, hard exercise, very cold temperatures and rapid weight loss, can bring on drug withdrawals suddenly. Therefore it is important to avoid these conditions as much as possible.

I had low tolerance to the side effects of psychotropic drugs, and was similarly sensitive to them as they were being released from my body. As these drugs were discharged from my body they mimicked the illness they were taken to combat.

At first the withdrawals were debilitating, but as time went by I was less bothered by them. I was taught by my Truehope counselor to remember that each time I felt bad, I should remind myself that I was actually getting better, that the drugs were leaving my body.

I managed the symptoms of drug withdrawals by drinking four scoops of flavored isolated protein powder every day in cold water. This protein, which can be purchased at natural food stores or supplement stores, was a life saver.

Protein isolate binds to the chemicals in the anti-depressants as they drop into the bloodstream, acting as a buffer and preventing further symptoms. In time I learned to recognize when I was having withdrawals coming on, and could act quickly to help myself feel better.

When I first started taking the EMPowerplus I was not aware of the dangerous and destructive effects psychotropic medicines could have on the body, mind and general health. Staying close to my Truehope counselor helped me to stay positive when I felt ill.

I had my last drug withdrawal incident in the summer of 2013, ten years after starting on the Truehope program. It was July, the hottest month of the year, when I suddenly felt like I had the flu. I thought it was unusual, and within a couple of days I realized that it was actually withdrawals. I immediately purchased a small bottle of protein isolated and within twenty-four hours I felt better.

Truehope has developed a new product called Transition Support which was designed to help reduce anxiety, improve sleep and increase relaxation during this difficult time.

EMPOWERPLUS

The micronutrient formula needs to be taken consistently, in similar doses and at regular intervals. I usually take the capsules after meals, and with an eight ounce glass of water. I personally do not like to take the EMPowerplus after 3:00pm because I go to bed at 9:00pm. It is very important not to take it later than 6:00pm because taking it later can keep you awake at night.

EXTRA MINERALS

No other minerals can be added to the diet because the balance of the nutrients in the EMPowerplus will be affected, and can cause depression to return.

While working at GNC, I suddenly began to get depressed. I figured out with the help of my Truehope counselor, that my new habit of eating protein bars for lunch had to be discontinued because of their high mineral content. This taught me to read the labels on purchased products to see if there were added minerals.

The Truehope BMD brand of calcium has been specifically formulated to work with the micronutrients, and is therefore the only extra mineral source which can be taken without symptoms returning.

GENETICALLY MODIFIED FOODS

These biochemically altered foods are proving disastrous to man and beast alike. They are causing serious digestive problems which are leading to chronic illnesses. I recommend that anyone having digestive problems educate themselves on this topic.

HYDRATION

I have lived in the western United States for over a quarter century and have come to understand the importance of water. In the summer I drink around a gallon of filtered water daily, and in the winter I still drink every hour. Drinking plenty of water helps with energy levels, detoxification and with the absorption of EMPowerplus.

ILLNESS

Truehope explained to me that when we are sick the nutrients in EMPowerplus are diverted towards the healing of the body. It is therefore important to increase the amount of EMPowerplus during times of illness to keep the brain supplied and balanced chemically. Always consult with a Truehope counselor before increasing or decreasing the number of capsules of EMPowerplus.

LEAKY GUT SYNDROME

Leaky gut syndrome is a condition where the small intestine develops inflammation and becomes damaged over time. This condition is directly responsible for a wide range of illnesses, including those leading to problems in the central nervous system. Therefore, the brain is affected when the health of the intestines is compromised.

SLEEP

I slept pretty well as a child, although when I was experiencing stress I sometimes had a hard time falling asleep. I began having serious insomnia after the birth my first child, and with the escalation of abuse in my marriage. My daughter was premature and I had to get up to nurse her every two hours of the night in the first few months. I developed anxiety as I became more and more sleep deprived.

The summer after I divorced my husband I could not sleep at all. After weeks of suffering I finally went to a doctor, who prescribed sleeping pills. I took one the first night and still could not sleep. I took two the next night and was up all night with a racing heartbeat. I decided that sleeping pills were no good for me, and threw them out. I remembered learning years before that a calcium deficiency can lead to a lack of sleep. So I bought calcium and took double the amount recommended. In one week I was sleeping through the night.

As the years went by and my stress level went up, I had a harder time falling asleep and staying asleep. After I started taking EMPowerplus I got into a routine of going to bed at 9:00pm. I found that I slept better and longer by going to bed earlier. If I went to bed late, I usually woke early and could not sleep in.

As my children became teenagers and started working after school, going to dances and other activities, I found staying up waiting for them to come home very difficult. I used to joke that I had just got them sleeping through the night, and then they became teenagers and kept me up again! Getting proper sleep has definitely been one of my biggest challenges.

● ● ●

SUGAR

I gave up buying white cane sugar after doing research into it in my early twenties. However, I have eaten a lot of sugar from other sources including chocolate, processed cheese, pastries, and jams, not to mention the hidden sources in other processed foods.

While trying to recover from gluten intolerance, I ate chocolate to help me put weight on. My diet was so limited and my digestion so poor, that chocolate became a staple food for a while. However, now that I have discovered my gluten intolerance is actually Celiac disease, I am radically changing my eating habits permanently. I now eat no sugar or alternative sweeteners and am feeling much better.

Sugar is a major contributor to the weakening of the stomach, small intestine and the nervous system. It is not really a food as it cannot be digested in the stomach, and passes straight through the intestinal wall into the bloodstream. It is highly addictive and a major contributor to stress. It is in most of the prepared foods in the supermarket, including cheese, and consequently, I have given up all processed foods as well.

STRESS

Stress is a major contributor to bipolar illness and it is important to do everything possible to lower stress levels. It has been a big problem in my life. I have been

● ● ●

stressed over everything from finances to how I was going to raise my children, to their schooling, to family problems. I worried constantly about how my children were handling my illness, and about my relationship with them. I stressed over what people around me were thinking of me, and about the ongoing negative relationship with my ex-husband. I stressed about going out to work, and whether I could work effectively to keep a job.

I now do everything I can to lower stress. I go to bed early, drive and shop at quieter times of the day, and if I have to drive long distances I take extra EMPowerplus and choline. I also make sure that I don't drive on an empty stomach so that I can be more focused. Driving long distances has been hard for me, probably because I was not raised in a long-distance driving culture. However, I am becoming more relaxed while driving longer distances, but I do like to take my time and break up long journeys.

For serious stress, Inositol, a B vitamin derivative in powder form, can be eaten directly from a spoon or added to a bottle of water.

SUPPORT

Surrounding yourself with supportive people as you go through this transition is a big plus. I had nobody to help me through it which made it that much harder. My main link to support was through the Truehope staff, and I am so grateful they were there. Having a supportive doctor or therapist is also very important, but I recognize that not all medical and psychiatric professionals will agree to monitor your progress.

WEIGHT GAIN

Weight gain from medications was very problematic for me. I was always thin and it was hard for me to deal with. However, I took Truehope's advice and just concentrated on getting well. Eventually, through food combining, I lost the excess, which came off very slowly and consistently over a two-year period. I had been on the EMPowerplus for six years when I started food combining, and five years later the weight has stayed off. It is important to remember that psychotropic medication is stored in the fat cells of the body, and fast weight loss can bring dangerous complications to recovery.

CHAPTER TEN

*"The sick in mind, and perhaps in body, are rendered more darkly
and hopelessly so by the manifold reflections of their disease
mirrored back from all quarters in the deportment of those about
them. They are compelled to inhale the poison of their own breath
by infinite repetition......."*

Nathaniel Hawthorne: The House of the Seven Gables

MY LIFE NOW

I'm going to relate an experience that impacted my
life for many years, and I shall have to go back in time to
emphasize how good my life has become.

As previously stated, it took me six years to
decrease the micronutrients to a maintenance dose, and to
get my thinking and behavior sorted out. My recovery was
definitely a process, and as each month and year passed I

• • •

felt increasingly able to function normally. My mental focus improved, and my ability to see things as they really are, increased. My physical energy and strength grew, and I felt more able to run my life.

Emotionally, however, I was still having trouble. In fact, in early 2010 I began to have deep feelings of hopelessness. I felt like I would never be a normal and happy person. I had been on EMPowerplus over six years and couldn't understand why I was feeling so negative.

I thought my problem was more of a spiritual one, so I made an appointment with one of my ecclesiastical leaders and told him how I was feeling. After an hour visit he told me he wanted me to go see a counselor. I was resistant to the idea at first, but I relented and said I would go.

I am going to recount the experience I had in therapy to show that healing from bipolar disorder is not just about balancing brain chemistry. After we are balanced chemically, there may be other work to do, especially in healing our thinking and behavior, and our relationships. There can be many factors at work which can impede our ability to get well.

Over the years when I was ill, and during the first seven years of recovery, I felt that I did not have the emotional reserves to make new friends and maintain relationships.

• • •

However, for twenty years I had someone in my life that I considered my best friend. She was someone I looked up to and trusted; someone who knew all there was to know about me. In time I felt that she was my only friend, and that I would never have any other friends. She seemed to be the only person I could really relate to, or who understood me for that matter.

It had been an unusual relationship from the start. She had put me on the road to beginning my healing work by telling me her own story of abuse. I came to rely on and trust her judgment, not only in personal issues, but in family struggles as well. She had become my mentor, my hero, often seemingly, my only link with reality.

In my heart I knew there was something not quite right, but I couldn't put my finger on it. She played the role of the all-wise therapist and I was the inexperienced, mentally ill and emotionally disturbed patient. From the beginning, it had been an unequal relationship.

Several times I had tried to pull away from her. I wouldn't call her for a couple of weeks, but she would call me and get mad, telling me that it took two people to have a relationship. I even tried to discuss my relationship with her several times, tried to put into words how I felt, but she always minimized and brushed aside my feelings. I felt I was in her debt. She had done so much for me and my children. I daren't do anything to alter the status quo.

• • •

For several years this friend and I had lived in different states, but we used to talk on the phone several times a week. Now we were in the same city again, first as neighbors, then sharing the same house.

When I first started doing emotional healing work, I believed in my heart that I would recover completely and live a normal life. However I was told by this individual that I could never expect to be truly healed, that I would have to make do with a kind of compromised existence. I could perhaps have a measure of happiness, enough to function and have a life, but I could never expect more than that.

Anyway, in 2010, thinking my problem was a spiritual one; I made an appointment with one of my ecclesiastical leaders. I told him how defeated I was feeling. After an hour visit he told me he wanted me to go see a counselor. I was resistant at first because I had spent so much time in counseling over the years. Eventually I agreed to go and made an appointment with the new therapist.

Meeting Kevin Johnson, who wrote the foreword, would become a life-altering experience. I went into therapy well prepared; I had started working on things while I waited six weeks to get in to see him. At first he thought I would need only a few sessions with him. Little did we both know what was going to happen.

After the first few sessions I began to feel much better, but as things unfolded it became apparent that I

• • •

would actually need to spend the entire twelve sessions allotted. I went into therapy to get myself fixed, but within a couple of weeks I knew that it was more than that.

Shortly after I started seeing Kevin, this friend and I had a disagreement. She told me to tell Kevin that I may be okay in his office, but I was not okay at home!

I was flabbergasted, because in the few sessions I had been going to therapy, I felt like I was making progress. I asked her to tell me what she thought the problem was. She dictated a long list, which I wrote down in a notebook.

I took the list with me to the next therapy session and Kevin looked it over. He then said something I never expected to hear. He told me that he had observed all those things after a couple of sessions with me; but he said she had no right to tell me any of them! He proceeded to explain to me why therapy and friendship don't mix.

The bottom seemed to drop out of my stomach. I felt an awful fear. I could not believe what I was hearing. My fear turned to disbelief, and then to sorrow. I felt like my world had just been turned upside down. Kevin saw my anguish and advised me to make strong boundaries with this person.

As he talked I began to see what had really been going on. All those years while I had been working so hard to make progress, to become emotionally healthy, this twenty-year relationship was actually the stumbling block to my becoming whole. I now see that ours was more of a

● ● ●

parent- child relationship, much the same as my husband's was with me; although I didn't understand any of that at the time. The glaring truth was that after my husband had walked out of one door, she had walked in the other. All my life I had been controlled by one person or another. I decided I would never allow it to happen again.

When I left his office I went to have a solitary dinner at a local restaurant. I mulled over what he had told me, and as I looked back over the previous twenty years, I saw all the times I had tried to extricate myself from the relationship. I would delay calling her for a couple of weeks, and she would call and berate me for not keeping in touch, saying that it takes two to make a relationship, and that I should be reciprocating. I always felt guilty, even though the knot in my stomach was getting bigger.

An hour later, as I walked across the parking lot to my car I suddenly felt happy. I suddenly felt something I had never felt before. I felt free.

As I drove home, reality hit and I wondered how I was going to behave now? I was afraid to face her. What was I going to say? I knew what Kevin had told me was right, but how would it all play out?

When I got back to the house I didn't know how to act, I didn't know what to do, what to say, how to start the process of setting limits. I was afraid of the repercussions. At first I tried staying out of her way, but that was hard to do.

● ● ●

Over the next couple of weeks in therapy I saw clearly what had been happening to me. My weaknesses had been constantly mirrored back to me, and my problems were regularly and consistently pointed out. After living in close proximity to her again, I had become horribly unsure of myself, and had a hard time being around her. I began shutting myself off in my room, watching television.

I became afraid to speak my mind, invite people to the house, or talk to my children in front of her. I felt like I had to watch myself, like I was always doing something wrong. In fact, she treated me just like one of the children. I was subjected to the same kind of treatment and scolding that the teenagers were.

I was floored, and had no idea that being under a microscope, under constant scrutiny, was eroding my self-worth and that it was this unhealthy relationship that was preventing me from being healed. This was the real reason for my feelings of hopelessness. Kevin told me that there had never been enough of a friendship for us to be living together. We were roommates at best, and she and had absolutely no right to do what she was doing.

This revelation changed my perspective, and I was changing along with it. It was like a massive spotlight had been turned on and for the first time I was seeing the situation for what it really was.

Life at our house became very hard. You don't walk away from someone who has controlled your life, and

● ● ●

every thought, for twenty years, without major recriminations and a massive backlash. This relationship was intertwined and embedded with many others, including with my children, and I was perceived as a disloyal, ungrateful traitor. Things came to an ugly head and I moved out. My youngest son, who had just graduated from high school, chose not to go with me.

As painful as it was to leave my son behind, this move marked the beginning of a new life for me. I knew I could no more return to a relationship with this person, than I could to my ex-husband. Unfortunately, neither this individual, nor any of the others closely interwoven with us, could possibly understand what had happened, or what was happening.

I knew, though, that I was doing the right thing, and that if I was going to make progress and become emotionally independent, I had to set about extricating myself from the intricate web that had enveloped every aspect of my life.

I felt very alone, and that I had no credibility with anyone that had been involved in our lives. One by one the recriminations and judgments started, and I sometimes doubted my own judgment. The whole scenario reminded me of my separation from my husband; it was like a divorce and people took sides-mostly against me.

I was entering a brave new world, one in which I was going to become the principal character in my own life-

• • •

finally. If anyone were to ask me why I walked away from this relationship, I would ask them why a woman with no friends other than this one walks away and doesn't look back. There is a reason that someone in her fifties leaves a twenty-year relationship; and middle-aged women don't make new friends easily.

It took me a few months to get myself sorted out after this traumatic time, but the changes I made, both in therapy and out, were permanent. As time went by I literally became the center of my own life for the first time. Within a year or so, my working life also changed radically through a series of miracles, and I became a writer and public speaker.

On New Year's Eve 2013 I moved to a little Idaho town. I was terrified to do so, especially when I was told about the extremely harsh winters. I didn't know if I could cope with the cold. I'd lived in St George, Utah, for almost ten years and was used to very short, mild winters. I didn't know if I could live and drive in the snow, and I was worried that I might develop depression again. However, I not only survived the winter, I enjoyed it, and did not suffer one ounce of depression-a testament to the efficacy of the EMPowerplus.

My life in small town Idaho suits me well. In fact I have been welcomed warmly and have made many new and wonderful friends. I now understand that it is not particularly what you find when you move to a new location,

● ● ●

but what you take with you to that place, that makes the difference. I believe that when we are mentally and emotionally healthy we can adapt to any change, as long as we are traveling in the right direction.

Over the past four years since that relationship ended, I have become excited about meeting new people. I feel confident and happy. Every day is like a new adventure, and I look forward to seeing what will happen, and who I'm going to meet.

I've discovered that I do have the mental and emotional reserves for new friendships. Friendships with men are just as good as with women, and I am as comfortable with teenagers and children as I am with the elderly.

Recovery from bipolar disorder has been hard, especially as medications complicated the healing process; lengthening the time it has taken me to get well. Nevertheless, I would go through it all again to be where I am today.

My life has a greater quality of purpose and I have found great meaning in my suffering. My desire now is to share what I have learned with others; to help those struggling with mental illness know that there is a way out of the prison that is their own mind.

As a child, morose, depressed, anxious and afraid, I saw no future. I never imagined that I would ever be happy-but I am. I am indeed - a very happy woman.

• • •

APPENDIX I

GENERAL SYMPTOMS OF BIPOLAR DISORDER:

- Losing touch with reality.
- Delusions of grandeur.
- Hallucinations.
- Hearing voices.
- Spending sprees.
- Workaholic.
- Periodic anger outbursts combined with cyclical depressions.
- Mania exploding into athletic aggressiveness and long high-energy workweeks.
- Melancholia may be seen as energy slumps from periods of hard work.
- Emotional roller coaster of highs and lows.
- Each episode can last hours, days, weeks or months.
- Episodes vary in pattern, length and frequency.
- Emotionally feels out of control.
- Unhappy, angry and frustrated because not sure what is happening.

• • •

MISSION IMPROBABLE

- In its milder stages bipolar disorder produces a highly motivated, self-confident person who is astonishingly creative, has great social skills, and can work harder than many. In its worst manifestations, the disorder can lead to uncontrolled anger, violence, and psychotic detachment from reality or suicide.
- Feel on top of the world. Not even bad news can change the happy feelings.
- Excited and restless.
- Intense energy.
- Can go without sleep for days.
- Have countless ideas of things they want to do in life or achieve.
- Believe they can do anything.
- Racing thoughts and rapid speech.
- Irritable and easily angered.
- May start fights or arguments.
- Easily distracted and rarely follow through with grand plans.
- Unable to pay attention to one thing at a time.
- Make foolish decisions and have poor judgment.
- Acts recklessly e.g. with money, credit cards, driving, drugs.
- Unusually high sex drive.
- Severe mania can produce hallucinations.
- May see or hear or taste things that are not there.

• • •

- Manic episodes may not be remembered.
- Constant thoughts of suicide to end emotional pain.
- Feel sad and empty.
- Nothing can cheer them up.
- Constant feelings of guilt, worthlessness or helplessness.
- Feeling tired and slowed down.
- Loss of interest in daily activities and pleasures.
- Difficulty concentrating and making decisions.
- Weight loss or gain without trying to.
- Aches and pains – hypochondria.
- Lose the ability to function in daily life. Spend days or weeks in bed.
- Suicidal ideation. 50% of all people with bipolar disorder will attempt suicide at least once. Some suicides are impulsive, others are well thought out plans based on accumulated despair of life traumas. Suicide can be attempted because of many factors – repeated stress; relationship problems; deeply-felt apprehension; angry turmoil; despair at normal life milestones not being achieved.
- One in 11 people in the USA will be affected by this disorder at some time in their life.
- Manic depression and depression are the most common mental health problems in the USA.
- With time and no treatment, the disease will exacerbate the episodes and they will grow more intense, occur more often and be less amenable to psychotropic medicine.

- 25% of overcoming bipolar disorder is treatment. 75% is learning how to handle or avoid stress.
- Other disorders which coexist with bipolar disorder are eating disorders, severe headaches or migraines, panic disorder and muscle and joint pain.
- Bipolar disorder can appear at any age-more and more children are being diagnosed-and it gets worse with age.
- Tends to run in families.
- Genetics, environment and chemistry are all factors. It is not a character weakness.
- Medications and illegal drugs can also trigger symptoms.
- Stroke, brain tumor, seizure, birth of a child, and other traumas can trigger symptoms.
- If left untreated it can destroy a person's life.
- Bipolar disorder can interfere with a person's ability to go to school and work.
- Difficulty maintaining friendships.
- Bipolar sufferers are viewed as self-centered and untrustworthy.
- Good and bad stressors can worsen symptoms.
- In 60% of cases the first occurrence of depression or mania is caused by a major stress.
- Negative life events increase the number of mood relapses and lengthen the time it takes to recuperate from a bout of mania or depression. If no major negative stressor precedes the relapse it takes an average of 4 months to

• • •

recover. If a significant negative incident occurs before a setback it takes an average of 11 months to recover.

- The more mood changes, the more vulnerability to setbacks increases and the effects of certain medications decrease.
- High risk of suicide when recovering from a setback.

MISSION IMPROBABLE

APPENDIX II

SYMPTOMS IN CHILDREN

- Colic in infancy
- Upset stomach and spitting up
- Excessive crying that sounds like screaming
- Wanting to be held all the time; or not wanting to be hugged or touched
- Light sleeping and erratic sleep patterns
- Violent tantrums
- Extreme shyness and fear of people; or extreme gregariousness
- Wants to be in control of everything
- Violent bullying of younger siblings and cannot be left alone with them
- Unpredictable behavior
- Intense, purposeful destruction of property
- Intense hurting of animals
- No or low impulse control
- Extreme anxiety
- Delight causing pain and harm

- High separation anxiety with screaming
- Don't like going to school or church – crowds upset them
- Incessant chewing on clothes and blankets
- Need structure and controlled, consistent activities
- Extreme and irrational fears e.g. of vacuum cleaners, balloons
- Afraid of loud noises e.g. fireworks or other loud bangs
- Socially awkward and have a hard time making new friends
- Want to control play with peers
- Withdrawn
- Fixated on things – possessions, toys, movies etc.
- Loud singing or shouting for long periods
- Extremely intelligent and tend to talk early or delayed incoherent speech
- Fixated on doing things and talk about it constantly
- Problems with motor skills especially balance – clumsy

- Intense concentration for long periods; or short concentration span – like ADD
- Screaming when hungry
- Food allergies
- Picky eater
- Controls through food
- Large appetite for preferred foods
- Poor attachment to mother – toddlers don't seek mother out
- Like to spend time alone away from people
- Prefer one on one – high sibling rivalry
- Nervous and upset a lot
- Never seem really happy
- Creative and artistic
- Love reading
- Aggressive
- Panicky
- Tend to play with younger children-can't relate to peers
- Unstable and unpredictable behavior
- Don't like change
- Don't like sudden changes or moves

These symptoms in children have come from reading books, talking to parents and from personal observation of children.

There are so many families suffering who do not need to. Young children can be difficult, but if their behavior is causing serious disruption of family life and if behaviors cannot be changed through behavioral approaches, then these children may be in desperate need of brain nutrition.

I understand that parents don't want to think that there is anything wrong with their children, and they don't want to admit that there could be serious mental illness. However, it is better to act sooner than later. I have seen children as young as two struggling with moods, impulse control and attention problems, which could so easily be corrected, giving great relief to them and to their entire family.

What parents must understand is that mental illness does not go away with age. Troubled toddlers become school bullies, have problems with their studies, become runaway and drug addicted teens and out of wedlock parents. Some even shoot their classmates. I know it may sound far-fetched, but problems in childhood which seem like cute anomalies of the terrible twos, can escalate into full-blown behavioral problems which eventually may require intervention by social agencies and the law.

• • •

I urge parents who are seeing unusual behavioral problems in their children to think seriously about putting them on the EMPowerplus. These micronutrients can only help; and improvements in behavior, mood and impulses are very quickly noticed by observant parents.

MISSION IMPROBABLE

APPENDIX III

TRUEHOPE'S LIST OF POSSIBLE LIMITING FACTORS

- Use of street drugs including marijuana, hash, cocaine and all other like substances

- Continued use of central nervous system altering medication (SSRI's, etc.)

- Current use of oral antibiotics

- History of overuse of oral antibiotics

- Use of coffee or tea including Chinese green tea (Herbal teas are allowed as long as they are caffeine free and not mood altering) and other substances containing caffeine

- Use of mood altering herbs (Ginseng, St. John's Wart etc.)

- Use of alcohol

- Use of tobacco

• • •

MISSION IMPROBABLE

- Systemic yeast infection
- Known parasitic infection or history of such infection
- Flu & other transient illnesses
- Immunizations
- Hormone Replacement Therapy (HRT)
- Fad Diets
- Use of previous medications which may have the potential to cause protracted withdrawal
- Over-consumption of refined foods like white sugar, white flour, soda pop and junk food
- Weight gained while using prescribed CNS altering medications or street drugs
- Disease of the bowel
- Persistent loose or watery stool (even if only once a day)
- Persistent constipation
- Irritable Bowel Syndrome (IBS)
- Use of laxatives

• • •

- Lack of regular meals

- Irregular or insufficient sleep

- Use of antacid medication (Zantac, Prilosec, Tagamet, etc.)

MISSION IMPROBABLE

APPENDIX IV

CONTENTS OF EMPOWERPLUS BY TRUEHOPE

VITAMINS A, Bs, C, D, E, H
CALCIUM
CHROMIUM
COPPER
IRON
IODINE
MAGNESIUM
MANGANESE
MOLYBDENUM
PHOSPHORUS
POTASSIUM
SELENIUM
ZINC

• • •

MISSION IMPROBABLE

BIBLIOGRAPHY

I include this list simply because I have found these books helpful in my mental and emotional healing work over the past quarter century. They are listed in alphabetical order of author's name.

Prescription for Natural Healing - Phyllis A. Balch
Healing the Shame that Binds You - John Bradshaw
Homecoming - John Bradshaw
Family Secrets - John Bradshaw
Creating Love - John Bradshaw
Hand Reflexology - Mildred Carter
Body Reflexology - Mildred Carter
A Brilliant Madness - Patty Duke
Call Me Anna - The Autobiography of Patty Duke
His Mouth Runneth Over - Ruth La Ferla
Toxic Parents - Susan Forward and Craig Buck
Blink: The Power of Thinking without Thinking -
        Malcolm Gladwell
Men are from Mars, Women are from Venus - John
Gray

The House of the Seven Gables - Nathaniel
     Hawthorne
Men Who Hate Women and the Women Who Love
     Them - Susan Forward
Bipolar Kids – Rosalie Greenberg
An Unquiet Mind - Kay Redfield Jamison
Touched With Fire - Kay Redfield Jamison
Love is Letting Go of Fear - Gerald G. Jampolsky
Stop Walking on Eggshells - Mason and Kreger
I Hate You Don't Leave Me - Jerold J Kreisman
Impossible Cure - Amy Lansky
Mental Health Through Will Training - Abraham A. Low
     M.D.
Selections from Dr.Low's Works - Abraham A. Low
     M.D.
Peace Versus Power in the Family - Abraham A. Low
     M.D.
I Don't Have to Make Everything all Better - Gary B.
     Lundberg
Self Matters - Dr. Phil McGraw
The Emotion Code - Bradley Nelson
The Bipolar Child - Papalos and Papalos
People of the Lie - M. Scott Peck
The Road Less Traveled - M. Scott Peck

• • •

A Promise of Hope - Autumns Stringam
From Mission to Madness - Valeen Tippets
Feelings Buried Alive Never Die - Karol Kuhn Truman
Immortality - Dr. Joel Wallach
Bonds That Make Us Free - C. Terry Warner

$1.00
of the sale of this book will be
donated to
The Wellness Fund
TRUEHOPE NUTRITIONAL
SUPPORT LTD
PO BOX 888
RAYMOND, ALBERTA
T0K 2S0
CANADA
(888) 878-3467
www.truehope.com

MISSION IMPROBABLE is available as an e-book
on:
Amazon's Kindle & Barnes & Noble's Nook

• • •

S. Deborah Fryer

THE ASTONISHING TRUE STORY
OF
A WOMAN AFFLICTED WITH
BIPOLAR DISORDER
AND THE MIRACULOUS
TREATMENT
THAT CURED HER

A PROMISE OF HOPE

By
AUTUMN STRINGAM

PUBLISHED BY COLLINS
AN IMPRINT OF HARPER COLLINS
2007
Available from Truehope Nutritional Support Ltd,
Amazon, Kindle and bookstores everywhere
Also available on Audible.com read by the
author

● ● ●